"Meeting Rebecca opened up my eyes and vision for what is possible when you mix education, motivation, and accountability together. The ups and downs of going outside your comfort zone was made a lot easier knowing that she was there to speak to and fall back on."

—James

"Rebecca was someone I didn't know I needed but am so glad I stumbled across. She was and is an invaluable source of motivation, advice, and guidance throughout my journey to a healthier lifestyle . . . Her energy is contagious, her work ethic is inspiring, and her results are so motivating! She once said 'You are disciplined; tell yourself that.' Something so small and maybe insignificant to others really hit home to me. I am disciplined and I am leading a better and healthier life because of Rebecca."

—Amy

"I find Rebecca knowledgeable, confident, focused, positive, normal, inspirational, and, if I need to pick her brains, I feel comfortable in asking her."

—Di

"When I finally came across Rebecca's workout videos, she was the inspiration I needed! She got me excited to work out and get healthy. First the workouts and now with the nutrition plan, I feel that my life is finally on the right track, a healthy track, and I'm so happy to have Rebecca."

—Faith

"In November 2018, I met Rebecca at a Fit Camp that she was running at the gym that my husband and I own, and I truly believe that God brought her into my life at exactly the right time. I had just given birth to my second baby and was diving fully into my roles as a mother and a wife; however, I was forgetting about the most important thing: myself . . . I can truly say that Rebecca has given me tools to be the best version of myself through proper nutrition, fitness, and personal development."

—Sarah

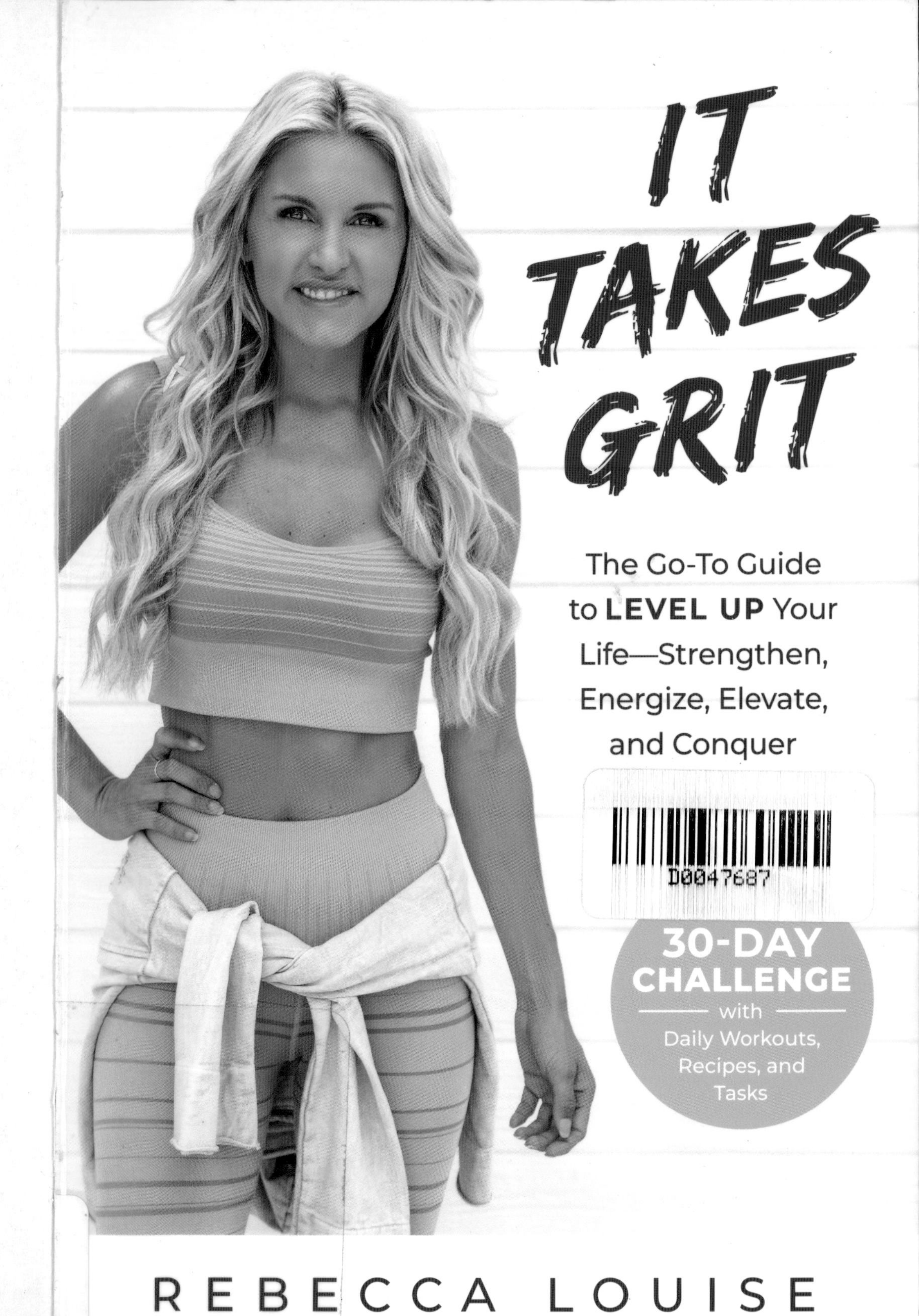

Client Testimonials

"This book is a game-changer. Not only does Rebecca deliver many laughs, but also messages in her stories that are jaw-dropping, inspiring, and they tell it to you straight! If you're looking for perspective on what's possible in life and how to step into your greatness, stick around and follow her lead! As my coach and mentor, her leadership has changed my life on so many levels and in tough moments where progress seems impossible, now all I have to ask myself is 'What would Rebecca Louise do?'"

—Meghan

"Rebecca has pushed me to be the best version of myself. She has taken my excuses and helped me flip my mindset to make them into action steps! Rebecca has taken the time and energy to become knowledgeable in fitness, nutrition, and mindset in order to help anyone she crosses paths with, including me. She is the definition of hard work and grit."

—Britany

"About five years ago I found Rebecca-Louise on YouTube and started doing her exercise videos. They were perfect for me as a mother who worked full time, and they helped me get in shape in the convenience of my own home . . . I no longer fear food, I am no longer ashamed of my past disorder, and I am in the best shape of my life as I approach my forties. Rebecca Louise has helped me gain control of my life, and I will never be able to thank her enough."

—Kimberly

"Not once has Rebecca told me what is wrong with me, rather she embraces what is RIGHT about the TRUE me. I learned to love myself. Rebecca has shown me that beauty is everywhere and in everything. She has guided me to see that life is worth living. Now I know the ultimate power within every moment, second, and, most important, MYSELF. I owe everything to Rebecca. Thank you for your deep beauty, inside and out. You are golden."

—Mo

"Rebecca has flipped upside down everything I thought I knew about fitness, nutrition, and business . . . Since Rebecca has become my coach and pretty much my lifesaver, I've learned how to take care of my body through fitness and the right nutrition; how to become a better, happier person through self-development; and how to set up my own business to help others do the same. I feel like everything I dream of is possible."

—Lily

"I don't know what magic this lady possesses but it has transformed my mind and body. It's not easy to get out of any rut or to start fresh with anything, but Rebecca makes you feel like you have an ally, a friend to back you up and stand by your side every step of the way. I am forever grateful."

—Heather

"Working with Rebecca Louise Fitness has completely given me a fresh outlook on my personal health and lifestyle. Learning to create physical goals and then actually achieve them in an enjoyable way has been so exhilarating! I didn't realize how damaging the formidable lies were that I had set up in my mind about my body and the way I looked. I hoped and tried to change, but many times I would battle questions on if it were actually possible. Now, after going on three months of following the nutrition plan and daily workouts, I can't believe my results. I'm strong and feel so healthy, and at the same time I've gained so much confidence about how I look."

—Lolly

"Having Rebecca as a coach has given me a whole new perspective toward life. She has educated me on nutrition and fitness, and brought so many positive changes to my life. She has taught me to be stronger than any of the negative things life can throw at us. She understands how it's healthy to feel the emotions that come with certain life experiences, but motivates and encourages me not to live in that dark space. I am so grateful for having Rebecca come into my life. She is inspiring and such a positive role model to me and so many others."

—Courtney

"Rebecca changed my life in so many ways, not just through health and fitness, but she completely changed my mindset . . . She's there every time I have a question or get lost in my own journey and her encouragement is endless! A coach is someone who believes in you more than you believe in yourself, who pushes you to be better than your very best. I am so thankful every single day that I put myself out there and made sure Rebecca Louise became my coach."

—Meghan

"Rebecca Louise has helped me transform my life in more ways than one. As a certified fitness trainer, I thought I knew everything I needed to know about health and nutrition. Little did I know I was going about it all the wrong way . . . She not only has helped me transform my healthy habits; she has provided me with the tools and knowledge necessary to transform my mindset. It is with her help and friendship that I have truly leveled up my results, relationships, and life!"

—Jessica

"I first started following Rebecca Louise through her Youtube channel. At the time I was looking to get back in shape while working out at home. I instantly fell in love with Rebecca's motivating energy, which made the workouts go by so quickly. This led me to joining her BURN app, which I am currently using to continue my fitness journey. Because of Rebecca, I have learned about living an overall healthy lifestyle and have seen amazing changes in myself both physically and mentally."

—Baily

IT TAKES GRIT

IT TAKES GRIT

The Go-To Guide to **LEVEL UP** Your Life—
Strengthen, Energize, Elevate, and Conquer

REBECCA LOUISE

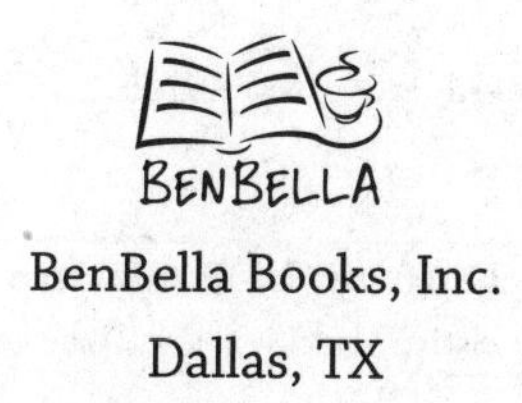

BenBella Books, Inc.
Dallas, TX

This book is for informational purposes only. It is not intended to serve as a substitute for professional medical advice. The author and publisher specifically disclaim any and all liability arising directly or indirectly from the use of any information contained in this book. A health care professional should be consulted regarding your specific medical situation. Any product mentioned in this book does not imply endorsement of that product by the author or publisher.

Exercise illustrations by Marina Federova, @marinafairy_art
Food illustrations by Janani Narahenpita

BenBella Books, Inc.
10440 N. Central Expressway, Suite 800
Dallas, TX 75231
www.benbellabooks.com
Send feedback to feedback@benbellabooks.com

BenBella is a federally registered trademark.

Printed in the United States of America
10 9 8 7 6 5 4 3 2 1

Library of Congress Control Number: 2020014050
ISBN 9781950665280 (trade paper)
ISBN 9781950665297 (electronic)

Editing by Trish Sebben Malone
Copyediting by Elizabeth Degenhard
Proofreading by Laura Cherkas and Cape Cod Compositors, Inc.
Indexing by Beverlee Day
Text design and composition by Aaron Edmiston
Cover design by Sarah Avinger
Cover and author photo by Cory Freeman
Printed by Lake Book Manufacturing

Distributed to the trade by Two Rivers Distribution, an Ingram brand
www.tworiversdistribution.com

To everyone who has joined me in a workout, supported me, and felt the BURN! I am forever grateful to you.

To my younger self for never giving up, endless grit, and to the person I have become.

Contents

Part III—The 30-Day Level Up Challenge

Acknowledgments

Let's be real: This book would not be in your hands right now had it not been for the people (and animals) in my life who have been part of this journey with me.

First off, to my dog Alphie, my sidekick and honestly the reason my workout videos took off in the first place. Even though you can be difficult at times, I would not change you for the world. I am so grateful that you sat on my mat, keeping everyone motivated as I worked out next to you. Not to forget my previous dog, Harvie, who appeared in the workouts, and my newest addition to the family, my sweet fur baby girl Pennie.

To my mum and dad, Joanne and Alan, who have always been an endless support for everything and anything I throw at them. Thank you for always having my back with my life choices, never judging me, and allowing me to be myself. (Not that you had much of a choice!)

To my brother, James, for endless banter, quotes from *The Office*, and for being on this personal development journey with me. I am so grateful that we get to work together and share passions, and that we are on the same page with life.

To everyone who has ever done a workout, or bought my app, nutrition plan, apparel, workout equipment, tour ticket, this book! I get to live my dream because of you and the support that you have shown. Meeting you all is the best feeling ever—thank you for believing in me and allowing me to be your coach.

To all my mentors, who have whipped me into shape, introduced me to personal development, and helped me grow. I am so appreciative of the time you have given me and for the community you exposed me to.

To my team of coaches, who are working together to help people with their nutrition and results. Together we have made a huge impact on communities and I am so grateful for all the memories we have shared.

To those who did not believe in me, for every single "no" they gave me. Thank you for giving me more belief in myself, teaching me grit, and making me step up my game.

To Cory, for allowing me to go for my dreams, supporting my wild ideas, and making me my breakfast shakes in the mornings. Thank you for coming on this crazy ride with me.

To my friends Danielle and Mel for telling me the truth, supporting me even when I have messed up, never judging me, and always being there for me. We have some wild stories for a different kind of book!

To all my staff over the years who have been part of building the brand. Each of you has had a role to play in serving the community; thank you for your time.

To Chris Winfield and Jen Gottlieb for seeing that I had a story and message to share, and introducing me to my book agents, Jaidree and Celeste from Park & Fine. Thank you all so much for believing in me; without this book I don't know if Mount Everest would have been on my horizon so soon!

And lastly to the team at BenBella Books, who took a leap of faith with me on publishing my first book. Thank you for seeing the vision. And thanks to my amazing editor, Trish, who did an excellent job of bringing my stories and thoughts together.

Introduction

Flying solo over LAX in a single-engine airplane at the wrong altitude was not my finest hour in the sky! During my flight training I made a number of errors—all that I learned from to become a better pilot. It's okay to make mistakes as long as we learn from them and understand we have a choice about what we do, who we are, and the way our minds can think. Good or bad, my choices have been my own, and my life experiences have made me who I am. With this book, I hope to share what I've learned and inspire you to level up your life, vibrate at a higher level, find a new state of happiness, and achieve things you haven't even considered yet!

Make the choice today that you will not just read this book; you will use it as a resource guide and handbook to take your fitness, health, mindset, and relationships to a whole new level of success.

What is grit? To me, grit is inside all of us. It is the burning desire to succeed that stops you from quitting and pushes you harder when times are difficult. Do I have doubts? Yes! Every bloody day. We all experience self-doubt, and I'm going to help you move past that and instill the belief in yourself that you need to keep going. Let's stop overthinking and *find your grit!*

If the same old habits haven't brought you the success and happiness you wish for, it's time to try something new. These new changes include your workouts, your eating habits, and, most importantly, your mindset. If you have *no* desire to add more value and impact to the world, then this book is not for you! Close it right now and go back to complaining, moaning, and floating through life.

Right from the start, I want to flip your mindset: The key to motivation is in action. Everyone is always talking about mind games to trick yourself into doing the thing! You will find motivation through action, because the action is what creates results—both short term and long term. With every result you see and feel, you will build more motivation. Don't look for motivation—it will find you when you develop the skill of discipline.

In these chapters, I'll help you find the grit it's going to take to get to where you want to be. By openly sharing my personal stories, I hope to help you see that struggle and failure are normal and give you the tools you will need to get through the tough times. I love the quote "Everyone wants to be successful until they see what it takes," and I hope that this book will help you discover that you *can* fight through it all and make it happen for yourself. If I can do it, so can you, and I am going to teach you the skills you need to find your grit and change your life! Let's do this!

PART I

WHAT IT TAKES

1

Action Before Motivation

At the end of the day, there are many ways to be successful, and no matter what success looks like to you, you won't get there until you take the first step. Discipline and motivation don't have to be things you're born with; they're habits you can choose to create. I have helped thousands of people change their mindsets and become healthier and happier, and if you make the choice to join us, I know you will see massive changes in your life, too. I am so excited for you to take the first steps toward discovering your true potential!

You wouldn't recognize the girl I was when I started this journey—in fact, you might have called me a train wreck, and even now I have days when I call myself a "functioning fuck-up"! You may feel like that sometimes too, and now is the time to put your big-girl pants on and keep going to get a little better every day. Girl, I am not here to let you quit!

One of the questions I am most often asked is, "How do you get and stay motivated?" I'm motivated by seeing results, which further inspires me to keep on going and to put my foot on the gas. There is no motivation without action, so just start! If you're losing motivation because you aren't seeing results or you feel "stuck," it's usually because you're not doing the work. Just taking one small step will break this pattern and move you forward. Each small victory will motivate you to take that next, bigger step for greater results.

One of the biggest steps I have taken so far was moving to a new country. Just because you come from somewhere doesn't mean you have to stay there. I think that everyone in their life should at one point live in another country to experience other cultures, create independence, and have a broader mindset. My hometown, Eastbourne, is a seaside beach town known as the retirement capital of England. It's a lovely town to grow up in, yet this was not where I saw my future. After seeing my first episode of *The Hills*, I knew that my life was destined for Southern California, driving down the Pacific Coast Highway in my convertible to a lunch date with my OC crew.

Seven years later, I finally made the move, and it was well worth the wait. It doesn't matter how long things take as long as you are doing your honest best each day. There were definitely times in those seven years that I was not doing my best, yet I remained focused on my big dream and committed to changing my negative behaviors to make my goal a reality. And while I may still be waiting for that lunch date with the OC crew fifteen years later, I'm not giving up now!

The first step in making this dream come true was a different approach than I had imagined. I thought my girl band (even though my mic always got muted because I can't sing!) or modeling work would catapult me to my dream life in Los Angeles, and instead my opportunity came through a new career option—flying planes! You may wonder if a family member was a pilot, or if I'd grown up loving air travel; the truth is simpler. I was living in London and had gotten myself into a toxic situation with a group of people that I needed to get away from. One day, when I was at my lowest, I happened to see a news story about a volcanic ash cloud in Iceland that had grounded flights throughout Europe. I watched a plane land on

TV, and I just said, "Fuck it, I'm going to be a pilot." Just before this revelation, I had experienced a crazy situation in London that led to the loss of friends and a job. It was almost like the ash cloud was in fact blowing away this chapter in my life. At the time, things seemed pretty awful, and now I see that they are actually fucking fantastic! A terrible situation led me to a decision that changed my life for the better, so now I don't see all of my experiences as "good" or "bad." Sometimes it just "is."

When I have an idea, I always do it, so three months later I landed at LAX airport ready to become a commercial pilot. I didn't know anyone who lived in America; all I knew was the hotel I was going to be staying at and the location of the flight school. The experience soon turned out to be less fulfilling than I expected—I was the only woman in the program and was constantly looked down on for not always understanding technical terms—and I began to wonder just what I'd gotten myself into. It would have been so easy to give up, yet I knew I still wanted to achieve my goal and get my commercial pilot's license. Around this time, I happened to meet an English guy on the hotel bus, and it turned out that he was studying at a different flight school. I went to check it out, loved the atmosphere, saw the opportunity I could have there, and immediately switched. It made all the difference. I didn't have to give up; I just had to make a slight shift!

On my first solo flight, I wasn't nervous until it was time to come into the traffic pattern to land. I realized I was 2,000 feet above where I was meant to be. As I asked the tower for permission to do a bunch of 360-degree turns to get to the right altitude, I started to feel my chest fill up and my shoulders get tense. I knew I just needed to get down to the right altitude and get into the traffic pattern. Ever heard of "survival mode"? In a life-or-death situation, you need to keep it together and focus on the solution. I held back the rising panic because I had to keep calm to safely land. I went back to the basics of my training, hearing my instructor's voice in my head telling me what to do, and because I had listened in class it was smooth sailing after that. It was only after I'd landed and taxied back to the flight school that I started to shake and think, "Oh, shit . . . what just happened? Am I ready to fly solo?" Maybe I wasn't, and when you find yourself at the wrong altitude (in my case, literally), you need to adjust and move on! Shit hits the fan all the time in life—controlling the way you react will solve problems faster, save your energy, and help you to grow.

"Change the way you look at things, and the things you look at will change."
—Wayne Dyer

I went on to get my private, multi-engine, instrument, and commercial license. I built up my flight hours and returned to England for my written exams, taking all of the steps that would allow me to become an employee of a major airline. It wasn't until I passed all thirteen written exams that I found myself questioning if I could envision myself in this career.

The answer was *absolutely not*! And that's okay—I gave it my best, gained incredible life experience, and then realized it was not for me. What I did know was that while life as a pilot was not my thing, Southern California, palm trees, and sunshine absolutely were, and I needed to find a way back and make it my home. Every step counts in life, and even if you feel like you step off your path once in a while, all of your experiences are valuable. When you look back, you'll often find that all the dots connect. Flight school didn't bring me a new career, yet it did bring me to California.

Now the bigger challenge was being able to stay and work in America! Thankfully from all my attempts to be in the entertainment industry there was some solid work that helped me get a three-year visa to work in America. As my visa was coming to an end, I had been dating my flight instructor for three years, so we decided to get married. For the first time, I was able to apply for a green card. We had a small engagement party and wedding ceremony and hoped to celebrate with a big wedding a year later, yet we never made it that far. A few months after we married, things went south and, ultimately, we realized we were not meant to be together. I flew out of the country for a work event five months after I had filed for my green card. I didn't think this would affect my application, as I still had my old work visa.

Turns out it did, and in a big way! Leaving the country canceled my green card because I had not applied for a travel permit allowing me to leave. I had no idea about this or what the consequences would be. I got the news that my green card had been canceled after the breakup of my marriage, and since we didn't end on good terms (and haven't spoken since the divorce), I certainly wasn't going to get any help trying to reapply for that green card.

I was struggling to quickly renew my work visa as I only had a few weeks before my time was up! As the time passed, I worried what the future had in store for me. I always believed that it was going to work out—it simply had to! Southern California was my home and I wanted to stay there. Ten days before my departure date I finally got the news that my original work visa had been renewed, and I was given another three years to stay in America. Close call!

During this time, I made one very important choice: My divorce and my visa troubles would not be an excuse to stop making workout videos and helping people get healthy. I would be crying, rocking back and forth on the sofa one minute, and then the next minute I would be bubbly Rebecca on a client call or showing you how to do a squat. No one knew. And there are still times when I'm not feeling 100 percent before a workout or speaking engagement, and I get my shit together and do it anyway. I simply don't make excuses once I've made a commitment. I made the choice to get a divorce, I took responsibility for the situation I had put myself in, and I made the decision not to merely continue with life; I was going to excel. Because I kept going, the month after my papers were filed for divorce was the biggest month to date for the growth and success of my business. Can you imagine if I had slowed down, let that situation get the better of me, or—worse yet—quit, just because times were hard? Hell, no!

We all have hard times, and we all have been in situations we would rather not be in. Yet, adversity is part of life, and it can't be an excuse to not push forward, go for your dreams, and level up! There are certainly times it's okay to grieve, bury your head under the duvet, or cry all the way through hot yoga where no one can see you, and then you will reach a point when you can either keep feeling sorry for yourself, or you can rise up, get out of your head, stop thinking, and start doing. We all experience adversity, so you may as well come out the other end with something to show for it.

10 Ways to Get Motivated

Experiencing divorce and having the uncertainty about where I would call home was not where I'd imagined I'd be at the age of twenty-five. During that time I was new to building my online presence and although I felt like my world had ended, I knew that to get out of the sticky situation I had put myself into, I needed to keep on working and chase my purpose. Along the way, I developed simple strategies for better health, a stronger mindset, and inspiration to level up my results, and I know you'll benefit from them, too. The following tips will set you on the path to success:

1. **Identify a role model.**
   It doesn't need to be a celebrity or popular figure—this person may be a teacher, friend, family member, or coworker. Find someone who has a vision for the future and is actively working to reach their goals. Attaching yourself to a role model sets a positive example for you and keeps you focused on your ambitions.

2. **Practice letting go of the past.**
   Go ahead and let it go! Don't dwell in the past. Take the lessons that you've gathered from previous life experiences and start moving

forward with your future. There might be a story that you are telling yourself about who you are that gives too much significance to the negative experiences of your past. It's time to rewrite that story of who you are to be all you were meant to be!

3. **Choose to focus on inspiration instead of doubt.**
   Whether it comes from inside you or from others, it's important to focus on what drives you without being held back by hesitation or fear. Whenever you start to feel doubt coming on, interrupt that thought with something that inspires you to keep going.

4. **Learn something new.**
   You can always make time to try out a craft, hobby, or practice to expand your horizons in different ways. No excuses—just decide to do something new and try it! Connecting with people can open you up to greater knowledge, so start by asking someone who inspires you about a part of their life that's deeper than surface level.

5. **Celebrate achievements.**
   Reward yourself for overcoming obstacles and reaching goals. You deserve it! And don't be afraid to share your personal successes with others—anyone who is bothered by you being proud of your accomplishments is not a person you want to have in your life anyway.

6. **Change at least one old habit.**
   No, really. Even the smallest things like flossing your teeth every day can make you feel that little bit of triumph that carries forward into other aspects of life. Take time to think about your negative tendencies and take action to overcome bad habits. I promise you'll feel better once you just begin! You have nothing to lose and everything to gain.

7. **Invest in good nutrition.**

   Your brain doesn't function at its highest capacity if your body isn't fueled by good nutrition. Your energy, morale, and creativity will suffer without the proper balance of foods, hydration, and physical activity. Eat the right foods to get your body and mind moving.

8. **Stop complaining.**

   Not only does complaining reinforce your negative thoughts, it also affects the people in your life who have to respond to this behavior. Do what it takes to remedy an unfavorable situation with grace, and if you can't change it, then learn to accept life's challenges. Examine your internal and external reactions to all kinds of circumstances and ask what results this behavior brings you. Whining is a waste of time—time that can be devoted to *thriving* instead.

9. **Move around.**

   If you're feeling stuck or in a jam, shake it out! Put on some music and get moving to change your physiological state. You'll be surprised how quickly the ideas start to flow. Sweat releases endorphins, which are going to make you happy, boost your energy, and give you all the good feels! You're never stuck; you've just stopped, and all you have to do to get "unstuck" is move. Move in any direction—it is all the right move!

10. **Remember what matters.**

    Avoid people, situations, and environments that take away your happiness. Be grateful for all the good things you have in your life and nurture the belief that things are not always as bad as your mind is making them out to be.

The first step in getting the most out of this book as well as your life is accepting that you have a choice—only you determine what you do. You might think, "I *don't* have a choice, Rebecca! You don't understand.

I have bills to pay, I don't have access to certain foods, and I don't have the connections to get where I want to be." Well, this is your chance to tell yourself that these situations are because of your choices and you get to change them today!

I know this sounds harsh, and remember, the purpose of this book isn't for me to agree with you; it's to change your way of thinking to live a happier life full of lots of "I can's." You can choose to believe that you don't have choices and allow your life to be dictated by that mindset, or you can try something new, work with me on the idea that you always have a choice, and see the results for yourself. The definition of insanity is doing the same thing over and over while expecting a different result. *Stop!* Stop doing the same thing, follow my lead, and let's level up those choices!

Task

- What is the story you have created about yourself?

  Write down all the events that have happened in your life—all through your life, the little things and the big things—that you see as being negative.

  Now take a look at that list, read it out loud, and notice that some of these stories have become attached to your identity, which in turn gives you significance, and this is why you hold on to these negative experiences as part of who you are. (For example, if you were cheated on in the past, you might be blaming that event for not being in a relationship now, holding on to the victim mentality that it will just happen again and using this as your identity and story.)

Now read it out loud a second time, this time detaching your identity from your words and merely listening to each item as an experience that you had.

As you uncover many of these events that happened in your life by reading them out loud, this time with a different meaning, you will start to recreate who you really are and get back to the core of your being—the *real* you who is not shaped by events that once happened. Your past doesn't have to be your story and does not define who you are today. Let go of those attachments to your identity that are stopping you from going further in the future.

2

Creating Healthy Habits

In my teens I made a choice to abuse and neglect my body through a lack of food. I thought that starving myself and living off seeds would not only make me skinny, it would also put me in control of my life, and therefore make me happy. I was definitely skinny at 86 pounds. Was I happy? Absolutely not. I am 5'2½" (yes, that half inch matters!), and I now weigh a healthy 105 to 108 pounds, so you can imagine how frail my body was at my lowest weight. Every day we make choices about how to treat our bodies, and so many of us make decisions that don't support our ultimate destiny and well-being. So how can you make better choices when it comes to your health?

Remember that your body is the only place you have to live. You wouldn't put water in a Rolls-Royce or neglect to fill up the gas tank, so why starve yourself or choose a nutrient-poor diet that is going to cause disease? Not only was my body suffering, my mental health was having an even bigger impact on my life. I struggled some days to even go to school or get out of bed because I was so unhappy within myself. Weekly visits to the doctor where she told me I was losing more weight gave me significance and inside my world, the phrase "You have lost more weight" was music to my ears. Now as I understand the damage I was doing to my body and the even bigger pain to my soul, those words strike fear into me. The thought of not being able to live my life to the fullest outweighs my need for control, looking a certain way, and holding on to my identity as an anorexic. Being able to let go of control was the scariest thing I had to do, and it was this letting go that in turn saved my life.

I am not a fan of fad diets, things that are just "in" right now and will be gone in five years. I'm a believer in the basics of good nutrition—feeding yourself high-quality, whole foods throughout the day, along with supplements to fill in the areas you are missing, to fuel your body and keep you feeling full. I also believe that food provides pleasure and social engagement—don't deprive yourself!

Identifying your reason and your "why" for getting healthy will also help you to make better choices. Ask yourself why you want to improve your health and lifestyle, and be honest. If you believe that being a healthy role model for your children is your "why," then look at them when you are about to make a poor choice. If you are still consistently making poor choices, then you need to look deeper for your motivation, because you either don't want to change, or the reason you've stated isn't enough to make a difference.

What motivated you in your teens will be different in your twenties and all throughout your life, which means your reasons for doing things will change. Visualize what it would feel and look like to achieve your results, and ask yourself: Why is it so important to get this feeling? This can help you identify your why. A great way I am able to stay on track and remain focused is by creating a mission statement. Distilling my motivation to one sentence that I can refer back to keeps me in alignment with my goals. Get ready to create your mission statement at the end of this chapter!

An online search about how to get results and make changes will provide an overwhelming number of options both useful and not-so-great, and getting healthy doesn't need to be a complicated series of fad diets and grueling fitness plans. The most important thing you can do is make the decision to start and level up so you can commit to it.

My destructive behavior started with an obsession to get skinny. I thought this would make me happy, and instead it consumed me every day. I knew I had to start again, so I began creating healthy habits to support my health, diet, and personal relationships, and these small changes became the key to waking up every facet of my life.

10 Habits to Improve Your Health

When I made the decision to change my life, my poor diet was the first thing I chose to change. Here are ten healthy eating and fitness habits to get you started:

1. **Eat a healthy breakfast.**
   Can you imagine waking up, starting your day, and not fueling your body to do the work? It's like trying to start a car with no gas in the engine; it's not going to move. Most people either skip breakfast or, worse, grab something unhealthy on the go. Starting my day with a healthy smoothie changed everything for me. Instead of cereal and toast, which are carbs that turn into sugars, my breakfast now included protein, carbs, and good fats along with a bunch of other vitamins and minerals. Suddenly I was no longer hungry or tired by mid-morning! I instantly felt better and more energized, and I was able to maintain my blood sugar levels. Eating a balanced breakfast within thirty minutes of waking up will spark your metabolism for the day, and you'll find yourself healthier and happier!

2. **Drink more water.**

   Get in the habit of drinking plenty of water and make it a priority in your life. Get a big jug or water bottle that you can fill up at the beginning of the day, keep it close, and get yourself through it. It's always easier said than done, and it's something I'm still working on myself. Proper hydration helps a great deal with weight loss and overall health. If you are drinking sodas (yes, even diet sodas) and lots of fruit juice, cut them out and replace them with water.

3. **Count protein.**

   I aim to eat 100 to 110 grams of protein each day because this is how much my body needs to stay full and maintain lean muscle mass. Your protein needs will vary based on your height, weight, sex, and goal (see Chapter 6). Hunger affects your mood, energy levels, and basic bodily functions. There's no need to be weak and grouchy, so determine the amount of protein you need and fuel yourself properly every day.

4. **Eat when you are hungry.**

   I used to fast after 7 PM, and I forced many ex-boyfriends to join me in this practice! If you eat at 6 PM and then you don't eat anything until 8 AM, that's fourteen hours without food! Long fasting periods such as this can put your body into starvation mode, which causes you to store fat. If you are hungry in the evening, go ahead and have a healthy protein snack—just avoid sugars. Sugars and simple carbs turn into fat, and not the good kind. They have little to no nutritional value and should be eaten in small amounts.

5. **Vary your workouts.**

   I played sports as a kid—field hockey, soccer, and more. I joined my first gym at sixteen and I had no idea what I was doing. Have you ever caught yourself staring at the machines thinking, "What the hell do I do here?" until you've finally stared for so long you just shrug it off and move on? Clearly, this method wasn't giving me any results, and I soon found that classes were a place where I could get the instruction and inspiration I needed. Mixing different styles of exercise, just like the fitness app I created, keeps me fit and balanced. For me, this is the key to motivation and not hitting a plateau, and it is why I have based my fitness routines on a variety of exercise styles.

Mixing up your workouts, from body weight, to kickboxing, to barre, to yoga, works different muscle groups and gives your body balance and a skill set for well-rounded fitness. You are constantly shocking your body into different directions and working on strength, endurance, and flexibility. It's overall health that you are looking for, not just a six-pack!

6. Give yourself rest days.

Your body needs time to repair. Have you ever worked out excessively and not seen results? Rest is a key element in getting results, along with nutrition and exercise. When you work your muscles, you are effectively tearing them down, so when they repair, they build back stronger and bigger. If you keep doing the same thing every day and working out too hard or without rest, your muscles don't have a chance to rebuild themselves, and you won't get toned.

7. Have a post-workout shake.

For a long time, I would go to the corner shop after my workout and eat a bunch of sweets. I mean, I just worked out, so why not treat myself with a bunch of yummy chocolate and candy, right? The thing is, although I had just burned a ton of calories, the reason I went to the gym was to get toned and see my abs. By eating all that crap after I worked out, I was trading fitness results for treats—all that work just for a couple of bites of something sweet!

Your body needs more than rest to recover; it also needs protein and the right ingredients to repair your muscles. When we are working out, we are breaking down the muscle and therefore need food to fuel repair and allow growth and change. Working out is 20 percent of how you look and feel—the remaining 80 percent comes down to what you put in your mouth!

A post-workout shake isn't just protein; in this case we need the ingredients that will repair our muscles and help us recover. Whey protein is considered the best for post-workout because it hits the muscles faster than any other protein source, which is important for broken-down fibers. A tri-core amino blend alongside glutamine helps provide immune support when you're pushing your body every day. BCAAs (branch chain amino acids) in your post-workout shake will help with muscle growth, and you'll also want to include carbohydrates to help replenish depleted glycogen levels. Most of the time you need to get these items separately to create the best post-recovery shake; there are some brands that have everything already included with the right servings. The one I use is available in my nutrition plans on my website (www.rebecca-louise.com).

8. Regulate your sleep.

When you wake up early and on time you set yourself up for a successful day. After a day of work, evenings are usually unproductive, so give yourself the best shot at using your time more efficiently by waking up earlier and going to bed earlier. I usually start to get ready for bed around 8:30 PM and wake up at 6 AM, and the only activities I cut out were unhealthy habits like watching television or scrolling social media. Waking early feels great—you can spend time by yourself with no distractions and enjoy some of the day before it gets crazy. Now, everyone's schedule is different; I get that. Choosing an earlier bedtime will eliminate binge eating in front of the TV and getting up earlier means you can spend more time reading, stretching, or just drinking a good old cup of tea!

9. Don't be scared of carbs.

For a long time, I thought carbs were the enemy and avoided eating them. Turns out healthy carbs, such as those in fruits and vegetables and whole grains, are actually a great source of energy that helps to build lean muscle. When people are getting ready for vacations or bikini competitions, they cut out carbs to get short-term, fast results. Extreme low-carb diets affect brain function, making you moody, tired, and irritable. Plus, as soon as you add carbs back to your diet, that temporary weight loss is gone!

10. Create a morning routine.

Making my morning routine a priority improved my physical and emotional health, and it will help you, too. Eating breakfast within thirty minutes of waking up to fuel your body for energy and focus is key to set you up for the next activities. I like to listen to personal development online while I get ready and then take fifteen minutes to read something along the same subject matter. Moving your body and getting a workout in before you tackle the day will help reduce stress and give you happy endorphins and a feeling of accomplishment because you've gotten some physical activity done! Check out Chapter 8 for more details on my morning routine and how you can create one for yourself!

At the core of these ten choices is one simple truth: How you look and feel is all down to you. No one is forcing you to have a whole chocolate bar or that extra serving of chips. Take pride in yourself, and level up your mindset by taking control of your actions. Do I have an occasional cheat meal? Yes, I do! And I don't have one every day. It is my responsibility as a human being and role model to others to stay in good health. It's your responsibility to look after yourself for you, your family, and our planet. Instead of blaming your friends' choices as the reason why you went with fries rather than a side of veggies at dinner, own your choices and take responsibility for your actions.

Goals are simply the daily decisions you make that create the outcome you desire, so make your choices based on the outcome you are seeking. The goal is not to lose pounds—that is the outcome. The goal is to eat veggies in two of your daily meals and get thirty minutes of exercise three times a week. When you implement these goals, that is when you will see results. Instead of focusing on the weight you need to lose or gain, focus on the daily tasks that will help you get there.

And yes, peer pressure is going to creep in from time to time, and sometimes you are going to give in. While an occasional slip is fine, if you are consistently straying from your goals when you're with your friends, you may need to do something about it. This might mean not being around those people anymore. If you are excited about your journey and they cannot support it, it's time to say goodbye, find new friends who support your goals, and move on. It's never easy. It's always worth it.

Creating Healthy Relationships

At one time, my only friends went out three times a week and stayed up until the sun came out. Even though I have always been a hardworking, entrepreneurial soul who loves people, I was never able to shine because of the environment I put myself in. I thought by leaving London I could escape the drugs and alcohol, yet as soon as I moved to America at twenty-three, I went right back to the same habits. My location had changed, yet I had not, and this is why I was still attracting the same behavior.

I haven't just dabbled in drugs. I have done my fair share, and there have been times when I have felt like I was addicted. There were periods of my life when I used cocaine by myself every day for a month—not to party, to just get through the day. As I look back now it's easy to see how out of the loop I was with life and how unhappy I actually was. All those lines of coke were just masking how sad and confused I felt inside. The way I feel today, feeding my body great nutrition and regular exercise with no drugs, is how I want to feel for the rest of my life. When I feel the urge to do something negative to my body, I have to remind myself that the reason I feel great right now is because of the happiness within me. Taking something to make me feel great is not sustainable forever. There is another way.

When I decided to make the shift to becoming a better person, taking my nutrition, health, and fitness seriously, those friends I had did not like the new Rebecca. As I sought personal development through motivational reading and lifestyle changes, my mind was expanding beyond their limited views. I wanted to follow the people who had dreams and aspirations and worked hard—so I did. When that group of friends disowned me, even though it felt like utter shit then, it was the best thing that ever happened to me. I did not know many other people in America at the time, yet I was prepared to make new friends who would support my journey to becoming better.

Sometimes I have felt like I am a split person. Half of me wanted to be a vegan, yogi hippie who sleeps on the earth, while the other side of me wanted to be on a yacht, spraying champagne and partying until 2 AM. It's okay to have these two sides, and I believe they can complement each other when you are aware. I love my incense, herbal tea, and meditation in the morning, and I can also go to a party and dance the night away with my friends. Life is about balance and getting to choose what you experience—you just have to ask yourself, do your choices align with who you want to be?

7 Healthy Relationships

An important part of balance is creating boundaries and being mindful of relationships you have in your life. It is key to acknowledge what your relationships are like and wake up to see what they are doing for you—good and bad. Here are the healthy relationships you need to nurture in your life:

1. **Food.**

   Feed your body good nutrition, eating a balanced diet with regular meals and snacks throughout the day. If you can't look after your own body, then you'll never be able to look after anyone else. Success in all areas of your life requires taking care of your health first. Fill yourself up with energy and wholesome foods so your attitude, mood, and behavior are positive for you and everyone around you.

2. **Exercise.**

   Are you exercising a healthy amount? You don't have to be excessive about it or push your body to the max—that's not a healthy relationship to have with exercise. Create an exercise habit by finding something that you love, enjoy, and want to do consistently. Exercise is crucial for keeping your body young—it promotes healthy skin, good circulation, muscle tone, and so much more. Try new things until you find what motivates you, then stick with it.

3. **Friends.**

   Do you want to be surrounded by people who lift you up or drag you down? The five people you spend the most time with are a direct reflection of who you are. Ask yourself, "Are they pushing me, enabling me to grow, and supporting me when I want to try new things?" Look at your current relationships and see if there is anyone you need to clear out to allow space for new, more positive relationships. Choose your five wisely!

4. **Your soul.**

   How many times have you compared yourself to others and felt like you were not good enough? If social media is affecting you in a negative way, you need to delete the people and accounts that don't make you feel good. When you're tempted to compare yourself to others, remember that social media is a cultivated highlight reel, not someone's reality. You are never on a level playing field when you compare. That person hasn't had the same upbringing as you, the same friends, the same experiences, the same education. So, what exactly are you comparing against? Someone who is nothing like you at all? The grass isn't always greener on the other side, so stop wasting your time.

5. **Alcohol and drugs.**
   Are you someone who lives to party every weekend? Or someone who likes to enjoy a glass of wine every once in a while? Remember that alcohol is a poison that slows your metabolism, makes you think differently, and affects your behavior and choices. Think about when you drink alcohol and who you drink alcohol with. Is it a healthy situation? Are you enabling your unhealthy relationship with alcohol or drugs? If so, it's time to make the choice to be better.

6. **Family.**
   They say you can't pick your family. I am going to let you in on an empowering secret: You *can* pick your family. If there is someone in your family who is being negative or is not a good influence on you, it's okay to focus on yourself and cut them out of your environment. Your family relationships can lift you up or bring you down. It's your choice and responsibility to do something about it if they are not bringing positivity into your life. Sometimes we feel like we have to be there for someone just because they are family. Remember, it's okay to cut the cord temporarily to take care of yourself.

7. **Partner/Spouse.**
   First, make sure that you are on the same page about your morals, values, and future. This relationship should be the most exciting one apart from your relationship with yourself. This person should always make you feel like you are the best person on this planet. Know that you can't change anyone—if you're expecting them to change, the only person you can change is yourself.

Take a moment to see where you are with these seven types of relationships. What are you thriving in and what do you feel could use some work? Write them both down—celebrating where you are crushing it and then what you are going to implement to make the other relationships match your best one. Nothing is ever going to be perfect, and we always have room to improve and grow. As you check in, remember that all of your relationships stem from you, the boundaries you set, and what you are willing to do to level up who you can be. Use the grit inside of you to find the desire to do the work, admit your faults, and change the things in your life that are going wrong.

Daily Habits to Wake Up Your Life

I have found that to have healthy relationships I needed to start by creating healthy habits in my daily life. This gave me the space to breathe new light into areas of my life that were lacking. From setting intentions to eating healthy and reducing physical and emotional clutter, these are the habits to focus on that will bring clarity and change to all aspects of your life. If you really want your life to change, it starts with making some small changes to yourself. I found that implementing some simple tasks for myself helped transform my thinking, productivity, and success in getting results.

1. **Set goals.**
   Each week, write down what you want to achieve so you can visually see what you have set out to accomplish, and keep this list in sight. Add the daily goals you need to accomplish to achieve the outcome you desire.

2. **Make a schedule.**
   Find a schedule that you can stick to, and do not commit to an exercise routine that you dislike. The ideal schedule is one that you

can practice consistently. Start easy: What time are you going to wake up in the morning? Really, what time are you *actually* going to get up every morning? Make it a habit by sticking to it each day.

3. **Clear the clutter.**
   Declutter and tidy your home and life. Get rid of everything you don't need and that might be holding you back mentally and energetically. Then tidy up your friends lists. Spend time with people who make you feel good and lift you up. Take a look each month at what needs to go, as part of making space for the new, good stuff is letting go of things and people that no longer serve your goals.

4. **Own your failures.**
   Everything good that happens to you is because of you and everything not-so-great is also because of you. Your failures belong entirely to you. Take it all in stride. Remember, failures are just the universe testing you to see how much you want something; just because you were not successful one time does not dictate what can happen on your third, tenth, or fiftieth time. Just keep going—you can't fail unless you quit!

5. **Seek balance.**
   Create a balance among time with family, friends, your job, school, fun, and personal time. There will definitely be times when you have to focus on one more than others to see the results that you need. Just know for a healthy, long life you want to allocate time for it all.

6. **Schedule time to reflect.**
   This can mean meditating, journaling, walking—anything that gives you an uninterrupted thirty minutes of self-reflection every day. Make it a habit, part of your daily routine. Filling your cup first allows you to be the best for other people.

7. **Reward yourself.**

   Make recognizing your accomplishments and successes both big and small a regular part of your life. Write down how you will reward yourself when you meet a goal, then follow through when it's time to give yourself recognition.

Throughout this chapter, you've focused on making solution-oriented decisions for your mental and physical well-being. The quickest way to fix an issue and move on is to focus on the solution, not the problem. Adopt healthy habits and create your routine. As you level up your thinking, you will learn to focus on finding the solution rather than dwelling on the problem.

Tasks

- Write a mission statement that identifies your "why." Be fearless, honest, and *specific*! For example, "My mission is to feed my body good nutrition and move my body daily so I can live longer and be a great role model to my friends and family" is better than just saying "My 'why' is my friends and family."
- Take a look at the 7 Healthy Relationships (pages 23–26) and score yourself for each on a scale of 1 to 10, with 1 being not-so-great and 10 being fantastic. This will immediately identify your first steps for improving your environment. Take action to get all of them to at least an 8!

3

Motivation: Why You and Why Now?

You picked up this book, which is the universe telling you that you are ready to take it to the next level and now is your time. There will never be a perfect moment in your life to start something new, so you may as well begin now. Give yourself permission to start and for it to be really messy! Yup, that's right! At the beginning it's going to be difficult, as you'll be dealing with mistakes, emotions, and new experiences, and that is true for everyone—me included. The sooner you begin, the sooner you can iron out the kinks and get to where you want to be. Get it out of your head that you have to have things laid out perfectly to start. We are all a hot mess at the beginning, so get ready to find your grit and figure shit out as you go.

Stop Comparing Yourself to Others

Are you spending time comparing yourself to other people? You are wasting your time! The biggest mistake you can make on your journey is to look left and right. Comparing yourself to others is only going to slow you down or, worse, derail your progress entirely. Keep looking forward, stay laser-focused, and keep your eyes on *your* prize, not someone else's. I know how hard this is—I compare myself to others and it can eat away at me when I choose to allow it. It can make me feel worthless, not good enough, and frustrated that I am not where I want to be. Let's help ourselves by taking a deep dive into the mindset of comparison and the steps to limit this unhelpful habit so we can focus on ourselves.

Their work versus your work.
Understand that it's not you versus them. It's the work you've done versus the work they've done. You cannot compare yourself to someone who has done more or different work than you. If you want their job, body, house, whatever it may be, just think of the steps they took to get there and do the same. People do not reach their goals by sitting around; they put on their big-girl pants and get it done. If you want it that badly, you'll use every ounce of your energy to make it happen. One of my favorite quotes says it all: "Everyone wants to be successful until they see what it takes."

When you're tempted to wallow in your feelings of inadequacy, try the following instead:

Be thankful.
Thank that person to whom you compare yourself. Why? Their success is proof that it is possible to achieve your dreams. Don't waste your precious energy wishing you were someone else—instead use that energy to do the work they've done without coming up with excuses. There's so much information out there,

so use sites like Google and YouTube to learn how to do the things you need to do. Find inspiration in the steps they've taken, execute the same steps, and know that it can be you one day who is the inspiration for others.

Embrace your journey.

Everyone has been dealt a different set of cards. Your journey is not the same as that of the person to whom you are comparing yourself. Everyone grew up with different households, circumstances, friends, and family. Maybe you've experienced a traumatic situation. Guess what? We all have—the key is to choose to not let your past determine your future. Embrace where you are now while pursuing where you want to be.

Be you.

You were put on this planet for a reason—you were born to be you! Everyone else is taken, so you might as well be the most kickass version of yourself. Embrace your uniqueness and shine bright! You have a responsibility to be great.

Invest in your development.

Take time each day to get into the right frame of mind. Listen to the *It Takes Grit* podcast for inspiration on how you can overcome any negative thinking, the worry of not being enough, and thoughts that hinder your success. I'm here to make sure you love yourself, reach your full potential, and stop wasting your energy wishing you were someone else.

Finding Your Grit

Now that you are ready to focus on yourself and your journey, you need to find that grit to stick it out for the long haul. Results don't come overnight; sometimes they don't come in a month, and whether you're building a business or even your glutes, sometimes it can take years. We all want immediate results because everything else is right at our fingertips. When we are going for our goals, we feel like we might not reach them, so we stop trying. Instead of quitting, why not keep going and figure out how to make it work? The only way to fail is to quit. If you don't quit, you didn't fail; it was simply a learning experience that you needed to have.

You are on your journey, growing and moving an inch closer to where you want to be every hour, day, week, and month. If you are not making mistakes, you are not living far enough outside of your comfort zone or pushing your standards higher. There is no need to live so carefully that you never fail, because that is a sign that you haven't really lived at all and right there you have failed. Go for what you want, and you'll come away with success, plus a bunch of stories and experiences you get to share because of it.

Don't quit just before you are about to hit the jackpot. Think of it this way: When you invest in your retirement fund (and trust me, you need to be doing this), you won't touch that money for years. During that time, your funds will go up, down, and up again. In the long run, though, the trend is upward, and you'll retire with much more than you started with.

You wouldn't pull out your money on a downward trend, would you? No! Your money needs to stay in the game, just like *you*! If you pull out when times are hard, you will never see the momentum and the overall success of yourself or your results. You need to play the game, be in it for the long run, commit, push harder in tough times, and inspire yourself to believe.

I promise you the universe is going to regularly test you on how much you want it. And all you have to do is keep on fighting, accept personal responsibility, and stay focused on solutions. Success will not just appear; for example, you have to develop the persona of a millionaire before you get the money. Think like someone who has the body you want before it happens to you. When I am having an off day, I look at myself and say, "I am not who I need to be personally to have the results I desire." Great! All the responsibility is on me, therefore what I get to do is work on myself, grow, keep going, and I will become that person I need to be to get to where I want to be. Don't be upset with the results you didn't get from the work you didn't do!

If you are not where you want to be, comparing yourself to others and thinking it's not fair, it's all on you. You are not the person you need to be to have these things, and now is your opportunity to grow into that person. Decide, choose to grow, and remember that things that come easy won't last and things that last don't come easy. Are you in it for the long run? Draw a line in the sand and say you are doing this *until*!

What if you don't like doing something? Don't give up because of it! There are going to be many aspects of life that you do not enjoy; if it is going to get you to your goal, you must suck it up and do it. While you have the full choice to say no, if you are striving for something that you really want, "no" is not an option.

If you are happy where you are, coasting through life, and not interested in reaching a goal, then I'm not speaking to you. Yet I don't think this is you, because you picked up this book to level up. So I'm going to tell you straight with no fluff: There are lots of things I have to do to get my life and business to a place that I love, and no one else is going to do them for me, so it's my responsibility to say yes and stick to my word when I want something to happen. The great news is that someday, when you've learned those skills and reached your goals, you can then teach other people to do the things you don't love doing. And you will never get to that point if you say no all the time.

I get it: We all need a break sometimes. If you're working hard 99 percent of the time, of course you can skip the occasional workout or healthy meal or say no to attending an event. Just don't say no to something just because you don't feel like it. Try to get through it instead, because it will only help you be closer to where you want to be. And, sure, if you are in no rush to get to your goal, or have no desire to even get there, go ahead and say no all day long! There were many times I didn't want to show up, yet I knew that if I didn't, I would be one step farther away from my goal of supporting my parents so they didn't have to work anymore. They were my "why," so saying no wasn't an option for me.

Just Say "Yes"

Use these tips next time to stay positive, keep moving forward toward your goals, believe in yourself, and do what's hard.

Not qualified? Say yes anyway.

The best way to learn something is by doing it. So, if you are not qualified for something or you don't feel you have the skills, simply say yes to the opportunity so you don't lose it, then go and figure it out. Most of the things I decided to do in my life, I had no idea how to do them first. Quick decisions often lead to opportunity and growth because you don't have the time to talk yourself out of it!

When I went for my audition to be on a YouTube fitness channel, I did not yet have my personal training license, and I had only been in the United States for three weeks after arriving with my work visa. Can you imagine if I had let the fact that I didn't think I was qualified or prepared stop me from going? I would not be where I am today, and you would not be feeling the burn!

Your past does not determine your future.

Whatever happened yesterday, last week, or last year does not have to affect the future as long as you don't let it. Spending time analyzing the past only sets you further behind. Accept the fact that what you did happened for a reason, it was meant to be this way, and it was setting you up for the lessons you needed to learn. Someone out there has done worse than you and has still made it happen—remember that. You can let the past control what you do in the future, or you can believe that both you and your circumstances can change and make the next part of your story bring value and impact to the world. Are you sucking energy from people, or are you giving light, love, and energy? Be someone of good energy, lift the mood, and always give back.

Find one person who believes in you.

We all need at least one person to believe in us. When two or more people have the same vision, anything is possible. All you need to do is find one person on this planet who believes in who you are and the ideas you have. Get yourself an accountability partner or a coach to keep you on track. No one can do everything alone, and with the right people around you, things can move much faster. Being around the right people is one of the keys to success, so if the group you are in isn't on the same page as you, it's time to find a new crew!

Create your burning desire.

Find the fuel inside of you that pushes you to achieve what you want. Strive to search deep down and find the point where you feel what it would be like to achieve your goals. How does it feel? Are you filled with adrenaline and excitement? No? Search deeper—you want to find the butterfly feelings that are buried down low. Believe unconditionally that this fire was put there because you are good enough to succeed and get what you want.

If they can do it, why can't you?

Why do you think you can't be successful when other people around you are literally showing you what to do? You are no different from those who have achieved success—they simply believed in themselves, surrounded themselves with people who helped to make it possible, and took massive action. Now it's your turn.

Do it anyway.
Stop making the excuses, level up, and do what you have to do. Don't let your reason why be your why not.

Dealing with Anxiety

Even when you have healthy habits in place, you won't always feel that you are in control of every moment. Paralyzing anxiety affects so many people, including me. It's hard to believe that you can lose so much of your self-control in an instant—from feeling normal, to feeling anxious, to a full-blown panic attack. The best way to deal with this is to forgive yourself for not being perfect, give yourself some grace, and move forward with the desire to keep on improving your reactions to the things that trigger you.

There have been many days when I just didn't feel like me. I would feel cloudy, out of breath, and confused, and I wished I could just sleep it off. I have arrived at restaurants to go out for lunch and physically felt like I couldn't leave the car, so I'd turn around and go home. Then, feeling even crazier because of what had just happened, I'd launch into a full panic attack and end up scratching myself until I bled to feel relief. Over time, I came up with seven actions I could take when I felt like this again without resorting to self-harm.

When your anxiety begins to spiral, try these techniques:

1. **Pinch yourself on the arm to bring you to a state of awareness.**
   Physical touch is a powerful technique to bring us back to level-headed thinking. A panic attack brings your mind somewhere else, and it's helpful to remind yourself that only you can control your emotions. I find that nine out of ten times a quick pinch on the arm can bring me back to reality and into a state of self-awareness, reminding me that I am in control. It is like when you correct a dog's

behavior by giving them a side tap to redirect their attention. Find a way to get your own attention so you can admit you are experiencing anxiety and then move on to the next step to calm yourself down.

2. **Slow down, breathe, listen, and move.**
   Once you acknowledge that you are anxious or having an anxiety attack and you've brought yourself to a state of awareness, you are then able to listen to information. Slow down, breathe, and fill your mind with something other than your own thoughts of what you think is true. Listen to your favorite personal development guru or use a simple meditation app to redirect your brain to positive thinking. As you listen to the words, repeat them, feel them go into your body, and you will start to see a shift in your physiological state. The power of positive words can change your attitude very quickly. Another great technique is to dance. It might sound silly, yet if you get your favorite tune playing, get up, and jump around, it will be hard not to smile. If you are somewhere where you can't just listen to a podcast or dance, the power of your breath is going to help put you back in charge. Take a big inhale through your nose, hold it for five seconds, and slowly breathe out. As you do this, allow your shoulders to fall away from your ears and start to smile. The goal is to have an action that can be your go-to as soon as you start to feel uneasy and worried. These techniques will help you to control the way that you feel, shorten the time you feel anxious, and eventually help you stop yourself from going over the edge into full meltdown mode.

3. **Write down the trigger.**
   Straight after you have done the above, write down what triggered your anxiety. It's easy to forget what made you anxious in the first place, and without this information you can't address the problem. Over time, see if you can identify a pattern. The key is not just to stop doing things that can set off your anxiety; instead find out why

you are anxious and what you can do to overcome it. For instance, if you get anxious every time you have to go to the gym, that doesn't mean you should stop going. If you did this every time something didn't feel right, then I am pretty sure you would never try anything new! Write down the reasons why going to the gym would make you feel great and then focus on the positive elements.

4. **Write down the worst thing that can happen.**

My brain is wired to immediately assume the worst, and before I know it I have fabricated a scenario that is not only unlikely, quite frankly it is often impossible. If negative is your "normal" too, you are definitely not alone. What I have realized is that when I look back, even my worst-case scenarios really aren't that bad. Yes, you might be uncomfortable, your tummy may drop, and perhaps you'll question what you are doing. Really, though, is it that bad? You are not in danger, and you aren't going to suddenly disappear!

Write down all the things that could happen if you do the thing you are anxious about, and if dying isn't on there, I have some great news! You are going to get through it. Plus, once you conquer the unknown, you will grow and be ready for more, and many of those things that seemed big and scary will no longer be an issue. Or you can give in to your anxieties, play small, and allow everything to seem such a huge challenge. It's your choice—get through it, do it anyway, and realize nothing bad is going to happen, or stay scared, be stuck where you are, and let every new experience cause challenges and roadblocks for you.

5. **Acknowledge.**

Put your hand up and say, "Yes, this happens to me." You are not crazy, out of control, or weird because you have anxiety. The quicker you acknowledge your anxiety, the quicker you can implement the skills to combat it. It is your responsibility to both acknowledge and have the will to do something about it. You are in control, and there are no excuses not to have this mentality.

6. **Have gratitude.**

   We can all choose to be grateful for what we have. When we strip back the busy life, the expectations, and the events we face, each of us is blessed to be alive. There is nothing that can't be fixed. I believe we can find solutions and see the good in everything that happens for us. Even if it doesn't seem like it at the time, I promise you will grow during difficult times. Write down three things that you are grateful for every single morning. For me, this puts the world into perspective and my life in context and helps me to enjoy my day more. When you feel anxious, remember all the amazing things you have in your life. If right now you think there isn't anything, you are wrong. Nurturing a victim mentality will not serve you or those around you. Choose to find the good and you will see it.

7. **Don't beat yourself up.**

   This takes practice. If your anxiety gets the best of you, acknowledge it and move on. Don't waste more time—you know what to do and you get to practice this again. This change will not happen overnight, so it's important to stay the course and keep working on yourself to get better. Quitting won't help. You are never going to be perfect, and that's not what you're striving for. Instead of thinking of it as anxiety, maybe call it an excited feeling. Start to implement the tools that will help you enjoy more of life's incredible experiences.

Tasks

- The first step can often be the hardest and the biggest one you take, so get it out of the way by starting *today*. What can you do right now that will get you closer to where you want to be? Take a fitness class, join the BURN by Rebecca Louise fitness app, start with one healthy meal, apply for a new course, open up a travel book to plan that trip, open a business bank account. It can be anything; simply take *one* step to get you moving forward.

- Find your accountability buddy and be very selective about it! This person needs to have high standards and goals of their own, calling you out on your bullshit. It might take you a while to find them, so start the search now and do not settle.

4

Getting Started: The 10-Step Mindset Guide to Getting Results

From getting into shape to eating healthy, being happy, and achieving success, your mindset dictates your results. If you level up your mindset, your path will be clear, and changes will happen quickly. Before we jump into your new nutrition plan and training schedule, let's get you thinking in a way that will set you up for success. Here is my 10-Step Mindset Guide to getting any results you want in life.

1. You Have a Choice

Acknowledge that you have a choice regarding everything you do in life. If you can't move past this concept, you will remain stuck right where you are. Surrendering to this concept will open up so many doors and allow you to level up. Reevaluate your decision making, find your why, and make it happen. Situations do not dictate choice; you do.

People are always telling me how lucky I am to live in Southern California. Luck?! It's not like I clicked my red Dorothy heels and magically appeared on a beach decked with palm trees. I used my savings to book a flight from London to LAX, used my legs to walk onto the plane, and worked hard from the moment I arrived. Make a choice to take action, let go of your thoughts about not having enough time, money, or resources, and just do it—you will find yourself "lucky," too!

Even if everything seems to be going against you, it is still possible to make decisions to say yes and find success. You *do* have the choice to make time to prepare healthy food and get a workout in. You *are* able to remove yourself from relationships that are no longer serving your highest purpose. And you *do* have the ability to take risks. Let go of excuses and make your choices based on the person you are seeking to become.

Are you listening to others' opinions and making life choices based on that rather than what you really feel inside? This is crazy! Only you can be the true judge of what you really want in life. If you want to get healthy and people are telling you that you are fine, think about the lives they are living. Is this something you want? Only take advice from people you would trade places with.

I may not have always made the best choices, yet I can look back at all of my choices as something great because they taught me something I needed to learn. If you feel like you made a bad choice, accept it, find the lesson in it, and move on.

Tasks

- Write down three of the biggest dreams you have ever wanted to accomplish. Next to each, write down the first step you would need to take to get there. Remember, you have a choice about absolutely everything and anything you can do. Make this crazy big!

  1. ______________________________
  2. ______________________________
  3. ______________________________

- Write down why it's important for you to achieve these three dreams and how you will feel once you get there. Remember, these are *your* dreams—they can be selfish ones. That's okay!

  1. ______________________________
  2. ______________________________
  3. ______________________________

2. Take Full Responsibility

Taking complete responsibility for absolutely everything that happens in your life, good or bad, is a choice that will put you in the fast lane for making things happen for yourself. Owning up to your choices and taking it in stride will help you to solve your problems quickly. The more time you spend blaming others for something that happened, the more time you waste. Waiting for someone else to take responsibility can take a lifetime. Owning up to it yourself helps you learn and grow. You won't make this mistake again, and you can move on!

When I found out my stuffed animal Pigow had inadvertently taken a trip outside the city of Madrid in Spain all by himself, my heart sank. At 11:30 on a Sunday night I found myself, age twenty-nine, ugly-crying at the front desk of my hotel, my face a mess of snot and tears, as I tried to determine the whereabouts of my precious cuddly toy who has been with me since I was two years old. They asked me to describe him, and I sobbed, "He's about this big"—making my hands about a foot apart—"he's pink, and he's got a little green jumper on." In my head I was also screaming, "*And he's never been to Madrid before!*" like that was an issue!

I remembered seeing him on the bed before I'd left the hotel earlier that day, and I realized I had forgotten to put him in my suitcase, which is how he ended up wrapped in bedding at a laundry facility somewhere outside of the city. Naturally, when life doesn't go our way, the first instinct is to blame someone or something else. I could have blamed the maid for not looking through the sheets, even though I know housekeeping's many responsibilities do not include looking out for little pink pigs! Finding Pigow was solely my responsibility, and I had to act fast to find the solution. As we've learned from shows like *The First 48*, those first hours someone goes missing are the most crucial! Because of my fast action and initiative, they sent a member of staff to the laundry place in the morning, and they found him. Phew! I was boarding a plane when I got the call he had been found; at this point I ensured that he would be sent via priority mail with all the tracking and insurance you can get. We were joyfully reunited the next day!

Find the solution. The quickest way to solve a problem or make a positive change is to focus on the solution. Don't you want to find a resolution as soon as possible anyway? Pointing fingers at everyone except yourself will only delay you in getting where you are trying to go.

Waiting for opportunity to fall into your lap will get you nowhere. At age eighteen I went on a train to London from my hometown of Eastbourne for a job interview, or at least that's what I thought it was! When I arrived at my "interview," I found a line of 4,000 other people waiting too!

It turned out that I had actually signed up for an audition to be on a TV show in the United Kingdom, a competition reality show for people who wanted to work in TV. While it wasn't the dream job I had expected, I decided to audition, and it was a whirlwind of an experience. I made it to the last week of the show only to be eliminated. As I came home from the last day of filming, more than a little disappointed, my then-boyfriend chose that moment to break up with me. In an email! I'd just lost the TV show, my world was upside down, I didn't have a job or university to go to, and I'd been unceremoniously dumped! Fan-bloody-tastic!

I spent some time wallowing in chocolate milk, self-pity, and shopping trips with my mum, and then I decided to take responsibility and get back in the game. I worked in a paper merchant to save money to move to London, spending each day literally stacking and counting pieces of paper on the 5 AM shift. I reached out to more than 100 recruitment agencies to try to get a job in London, and only one replied. One is all you need, though, and I got three interviews to work in banking, smashed them all, and got all three offers. I even fell down the stairs at my interview at Bloomberg and thought I had broken my knee! I moved to London with a great job and found myself living right next door to my ex, who surely thought I was stalking him. *Hey, neighbor!*

Don't blame anyone. Blame gets you nowhere fast. You can try all day, week, or month to get someone else to accept blame, or you can just take it yourself in a split second and move on. Which is better for your energy and soul? It doesn't have to mean you were right and they were wrong. Life is short! Accept what happened, take responsibility for your part, and move along. Be the bigger person, take a deep breath, count to ten, accept responsibility, and walk on.

Things begin to happen for you when you take 100 percent responsibility. During my career, I've had countless managers. Even though it is their job to find you work, be on your team, and help you to succeed, you can't just sign a contract, cross your fingers, and expect opportunities to magically appear. I've been dropped by at least seven managers over time, and each time I thought my whole career had fallen apart. Instead of giving up, I just told myself that they were not right for the path I was on. It didn't mean I wasn't good enough—if anything, I told myself *they* were not good enough and it was the universe putting me on a better path.

Rejection puts a knife in your heart and makes your stomach drop, and nobody likes feeling like crap. Each time I was dropped I took more and more responsibility that I was just not the right fit for them, and I simply needed to prove myself more to the industry. So instead of getting sad or annoyed, or, worse, quitting, I just worked harder. No one can take away your hard work, dedication, and resilience, so I leveled up my actions to do more. As you go through life, expect a ton of people not to believe in you. Take ownership of that and embrace it! Can you imagine if I had listened to some of the negativity I encountered?

"We don't know where we would place you in the industry; we can't see where you would fit." Funny now, seeing how I do fit in pretty well. People are not always right!

"You don't have enough followers and fan base to have an app." Excuse me?! I went on and built it anyway—your loss on 20 percent commission!

"There is no work for you. We've looked through all the emails from potential job offers and there's nothing there." I begged to differ and went back through the offers, taking the initiative and responsibility to follow up with them all. I ended up converting one to a job worth $30,000! Yeah really, nothing there!

"We are parting ways; this is our thirty days' notice." This was an unexpected email, with no explanation as to why I was being dropped! I suspect it was because I stopped paying them for public relations after spending $15,000 and not getting anything in return. They insisted they had never received one email inquiry, yet as soon as we switched my YouTube channel to my email address, the job proposals came rolling in.

And my all-time favorite: "*You aren't ready for a tour—we base this on how long people take selfies with you at your last meet-up!*"

Never think someone is doing all they can for you—the only person who can do all they can is *you*! You are in control of leveling up your responsibility for your career and life and making shit happen.

Does rejection like this sound familiar to you? Have you been told that something isn't possible for you? Don't listen! I honestly believe anyone can do anything when they make the right choices, take responsibility, and level up. As you can see, I didn't let someone else's opinion of me become my reality.

I built my career on grit and determination with no partners or investors. Just me. I searched for the right people to work with me who supported my vision. I have also worked with many people to find the few worth sticking with, and it only happened because I kept on going. Keep on going for *you* and take responsibility for making your own moves without relying on other people.

You are in control of your successes and failures. It's true—as I said before, everything good that happens to you is because of you, and everything not-so-great is because of you, too. Don't let other people take credit for your success! It was you who got there by making the right choices and taking responsibility for your actions. Your failures are also all yours. It's good to fail over and over and over again—it is all part of the process. Own your failures, figure out why you failed, and you will get ahead much more quickly. Remember that failures are just the universe testing you to see how much you want something.

Own your mistakes and learn from them. I'm going to let you in on something huge: The more mistakes you make, the further you will go. And the quicker you make all these mistakes, the quicker you will progress. No one ever got anywhere by doing things right all the time. You want to collect a whole bunch of mistakes, use them as life experiences, grow from them, and implement change. We don't grow by experiencing only pure bliss and happiness; we grow from the tough times. When something difficult is happening for you, embrace the mindset of, "Yes, this is great—I get to grow, learn, and level up." During difficult times, I always know that something great is on the other side, and I immediately begin to imagine what the universe has in store for me later when I pass this test. Take responsibility, level up, and get through it.

Tasks

- Think of three things that have happened to you in the last three months and take 100 percent responsibility for them. Go back and think about how it would have been much less time consuming for you to simply take them on yourself as your mistakes and learn from them.

- Call someone whom you have blamed in the past and apologize. While this is not an easy task, what you will get from it is going to be absolutely liberating. The feeling you will have afterward will give you so much adrenaline because you'll know you dropped your ego and leveled up to a whole new standard.

3. Remove All Excuses

Taking responsibility means eliminating excuses for why you are not doing something or behaving a certain way. Come up to me in person and try giving me an excuse, and let's see how that goes down! Each time you tell yourself why you can't do something, change your physiological state by moving your body, recognizing that you're making excuses, and do it anyway.

Don't let your reason "why" be your "why not." Let's say that you want something for your children or your family. You want to become a better person or grow your business or see fitness results, so you go to a trainer to learn how to do that. Then, at the same time, you use the excuse that you don't want to take time away from your family to achieve your goals, making your reason "why" the excuse for not doing the things you want to do *for them*! Taking time away from your family to grow and become better is not a bad thing at all! You are doing it for you *and* them. Wouldn't you want them to do it for themselves? Lead by example. Stop saying that you can't go to the gym, build your business, or do that thing (whatever it may be!) because you don't want to leave your kids or family. You need to go so you can be a healthy role model for them.

It was the night before Thanksgiving, and I was due to leave the apartment I could no longer afford that I had shared with my at the time soon-to-be-ex-husband. I was exhausted from packing and dealing with emotional strain, and I had missed my flight back to the United Kingdom. I spent my last night in that apartment on a sleeping bag with my dog, Alphie, and my wedding dress lying next to me. It was up there with the top shit nights I've ever had, feeling disconnected with the world and in my own bubble. I had lost my home, my circle of influence, and a husband, who also took my other dog Harvie, all overnight, and I lay there knowing that this was the first day of my new life. I had realized that I could not be with someone who didn't want to grow with me, who was content with the status quo, who rejected personal development and didn't like the idea of setting goals and leading from the front. When I made the decision that this was truly what I wanted without excuses, I felt free. Never settle! Nobody's perfect, yet if you are not fired up about the next year with your partner, how will you become the best version of you and reach your full potential? The truth is you won't, and it's better to be on your own than with someone who doesn't align with your values. Make no excuses for the person you are with.

Prioritize. If you really want something, it's at the top of your list. Be honest with yourself about what you really want to achieve in life. Are you serious about changing your eating and exercise habits, or just hoping to lose some pounds? Do you have a deep desire to have your own side hustle so you can have more income for your family? Whatever it is, do you really want it? If the answer is yes, all you have to do is make that a priority and eliminate the excuses that are stopping you from getting there.

Have you ever had a moment when the last thing you want to do is the thing you *must* do? Your brain searches for all the reasons why you shouldn't do it. It comes up with endless excuses that you are ready to list to anyone who will listen. Yep, I hear you. It's at those times when we don't want to show up that we have to the most. Force yourself to show up, because you will grow and level up the most in those moments.

Five minutes before I was due to give an important presentation, my dad called to tell me that my mum's dad, my granddad, had passed away. He was a real character, and I feel much of my grit, determination, and belief in myself have been inspired by him. He even made all the entrepreneurial mistakes for me by going bankrupt more than ten times trying to build different businesses and ideas!

Granddad had been hanging on for dear life, literally, as my mum and brother made it across thousands of miles to say goodbye. My mum landed just six hours after he passed away, and my dad let me know she hadn't made it in time. The loss of my granddad and the thought of my mum and brother being upset was heartbreaking. I had two minutes before I went onstage, and I made the quick decision that I was going to do what I was brought here for.

I was building a business to support my family, and they were my reason "why," so I didn't let this become my "why not" or an excuse not to carry out what I needed to do that day.

All excuses have the same value. Reason with yourself all day and you will be able to come up with the most wonderful and elaborate excuses why you can't do the things you want or need to do. The bottom line is that all, yes, *all* excuses have the same value: *zero*. When you allow some excuses to be more acceptable than others you will constantly be unsure. My goal here is to get you to understand you can't prioritize excuses. When you remove them all, no matter your circumstances, you will get to where you want to be. Yes, sad things happen. Either make something positive out of it, or dwell in the situation and bring yourself down. Life is so amazing, and we should be incredibly grateful to be alive. Don't waste opportunities and experiences because you feel your excuse is valid. It's not—none of them are! Embracing this mindset removes all obstacles and will get you exactly where you want to be!

Increase your confidence through action. Anyone else lack confidence sometimes? Yes! Everyone does. The only difference between you and that person out there who is beaming with confidence is that they have taken action to gain that confidence. If you aren't living up to your potential and meeting your goals, just start doing the things you want to do! Walking into a workout class the first time can be so daunting—you might worry that it will be difficult, or you won't know what equipment you need, or maybe even that others will judge you for your lack of experience. Once you have been two or three times, there is a level of comfort you have created because you know what to expect. Your confidence is higher because you have pushed through the first couple of classes, and you realize that most people are too busy focusing on what they are doing to even think about you. Stick with it, even if you don't succeed at first. Quitting after the first time is going to send you further away from reaching your goal.

Living in a foreign country has certainly challenged me. My family and best friend are a twelve-hour plane ride away, and I often have to watch my typically British sarcastic tone! It would have been easy for me to give up so many times, yet I never let excuses get the best of me. When the "why" is big enough, the "how" is easy. Regardless of the difficulties I've experienced as a British citizen, from buying a home, to setting up a business, to navigating taxes and medical insurance, I was still able to figure it all out without making excuses or giving up.

Don't have the time, the resources, the money, the confidence, the contacts, the education? These are just a figment of your imagination and the more you allow these excuses to hold you back, the more insurmountable they seem. Break the mold and think outside of the box. In a world full of instant access to information, ignorance is a choice. You can Google how to do absolutely anything these days. I never used the excuse "I don't know how to do it" to not do it. Read, watch YouTube, Google it, and figure it out—it's all there. You owe it to yourself to push past your excuses and begin living your dreams.

Tasks

- Write down every excuse you had in your head for the last three days, cross them out, and next to each write "All excuses have the same value."

- Next to where you wrote about your dreams from your Step 1 tasks (page 43), write down the excuses you have been making about why you haven't done these things yet. Then, stand up. Yes, get up and shake your body out. Reach up as high as you can, then reach a little farther and shout, "*Yes, I can do it!*" See how your body and mindset change when you feel the encouragement of your words in your body! Acknowledge that excuses prevent you from reaching your goals.

4. Control Your Reactions

How we react to something is often more important than the original event itself. My 100/0 rule of taking 100 percent responsibility while making 0 excuses helps me to react in a positive way. To help you decide if a conflict is worth your time, ask yourself if you are going to remember the details. Half the time we can't even remember what the original argument was about or what set us off in the first place.

I haven't always followed this rule myself. Whether getting in a taxi at 1 AM after many cocktails to chase an ex-boyfriend, taking it personally when my staff would leave, or panicking over issues with my app, I have had my moments of meltdowns and crying. I eventually realized that all businesses have staff turnover, products will be misdelivered, apps will break, we have all had one too many cocktails, and the only choice is to focus on solving the problem.

Maybe you've experienced that feeling in your gut that nothing will ever be right for you. Perhaps because you didn't get to the gym that day and you had an extra cookie, or you might have had a lazy day and not hustled for your business and are now feeling super guilty about it. These setbacks happen to everyone sometimes. The biggest comeback is how you deal with it and what you can learn from it.

If no one has ever said anything negative to you either online or in person, then you have not had your ears and eyes open. We all receive negativity in this increasingly online world, and we get to decide how we deal and react to it. Sure, you can fight back, argue, and defend yourself, which may boost your ego and get your adrenaline going. Or you can simply use this energy for something productive, let the opinions of others go, and move on with your life. If you know what they are saying is not true, why are you even allowing it space in your brain? Someone else's opinion of you is none of your business!

The more negativity you get online, the more positivity you're also going to get. I've heard that I'm too skinny, and I've also heard that I'm too muscular, and everything else in between. I've been told I'm too sarcastic (I'm British and this is how we talk). I don't take offense, and you shouldn't either. You can't please everyone, and your aim shouldn't be to do so.

For eight years my mum wanted this very special Louis Vuitton bag. After doing some extra work outside of her regular job as a head teacher she saved up the money to buy it. When she finally went to the store, it had gone up £50. She didn't have enough money, and the sales attendant didn't make her feel very good about that. Over the years my mum would post a picture of this bloody bag in our family group chat. I knew that one day I would have enough money to get it for her.

She came to meet me on a trip in Houston, Texas, and I thought that would be the perfect time to surprise her with this bag she had always wanted. Being able to turn up with that bag and see her reaction was one of the best moments of my life. We didn't come from money, we are not flashy, and material things are not important to us. The story of this bag and how long she had wanted it was what made it special, not the actual bag itself. After we got back to California, we visited the Louis Vuitton store, where I had explained what had happened all those years ago, and the staff made her feel so special that she broke down in tears.

The attendant in that first shop had the choice of how to react to a customer. Maybe he was having a bad day and took it out on my mum. Often your first impulse isn't the one you should lead with. Take a hot second to think about everything. The decisions you make today affect others and will shape your tomorrow. Here's how I do it:

Tips to Regain Control

Pinch yourself to bring yourself into a state of awareness. Often, we need to bring ourselves back into reality and out of the state of mind we have put ourselves in. Pinch yourself on the arm to bring yourself back to rational thinking and a clear mindset, and keep your mouth closed.

Take ten really long, deep breaths—then get moving.
Focus on each breath to slow down your movements. Do twenty squats or go for a run to divert your attention and get distracted.

Don't say anything back for at least an hour.
Hold your thoughts, allow your brain to calm down, and take time to react to events. You will have a much better resolution when you have not been immediately affected. Put your phone away or remove yourself from the situation. Speak to an unbiased person and see it from their point of view, which isn't easy *at all*. Yet it is crucial to you calming down and not taking it personally.

Solve the problem rather than argue your case.
Go straight to being solution-oriented rather than looking for someone to blame. React quickly in a positive way to get things fixed faster!

Ask yourself if you are going to remember the details.
Half the time we can't even remember what the original argument was about or what set us off in the first place. When issues seem so big, take some time to reflect afterward and ask yourself if it really matters in the long run. Usually, it doesn't.

Tasks

- Make a poster of the "Tips to Regain Control" (pages 54–55) and hang it on a wall where you can see it. Go through the steps to help train your brain whenever you need to rethink your reactions.

- Write down moments you've reacted poorly in the past. Identify the moment you could have caught yourself from stepping over the line and instead taken control.

5. Love Yourself

We've all been in situations where we've done things we didn't want to do or accepted less than what we deserve. Loving yourself means speaking up for your needs, forgiving yourself for your mistakes, and taking the time to care for your physical and emotional needs. It's so important to show up for yourself!

I have been in situations where I didn't want to have sex, and worried that the guy would lose interest in me if I didn't. Finding the strength to say no can be hard—the first time I said I just wanted to cuddle, the guy I was with got angry and accused me of getting him "all worked up," then put his clothes on and stormed out. I'm glad I didn't stick around for more of that relationship magic! You can say no, and you should if you have even a small doubt in your mind. Never let anyone tell you that it's not up to you to wait until you are ready, whenever that might be. If they don't like it, he or she is not your person.

Use the bad things that happen to you as a good way to grow. Feel blessed that you were able to experience something new and tap into that experience and what you can learn from it. Receive times of struggle, negativity, and difficulty with open arms. For every new experience you have, both good and bad, you learn something new and you receive a greater understanding of your emotions. You were dealt these cards for you to grow and level up, because the world saw more in you. So embrace it.

Don't beat yourself up when you have a bad day or make a mistake. We are all human, and mistakes are a part of life. Forgive yourself and move on! Don't you feel worse when you have let something you've done linger on in your mind for days? You can't change the past, and the more time you spend hating yourself for something you've done, the worse you are going to feel. Rather than obsessing about it, tell yourself that was the lesson you had to learn to move on to the next chapter. Make note of your feelings and reactions to help break that pattern of behavior in the future.

When your gut tells you something isn't right, trust that feeling. Shortly after passing my driver's test at seventeen years old, I answered an online ad for car promotion girls. Imagine my excitement—this would be the start of my modeling career, my gateway to *Vogue* (which I did appear in seven years later!), and the beginning of my catwalk career in Milan! It turned out, though, that this was not going to be my pathway to stardom, and in fact would be my first interaction with a pedophile. Brilliant, and on my first casting too!

When I was directed to a hotel room rather than the big casting room I'd seen on *America's Next Top Model*, I thought this was a little strange. I was so excited in my huge, boob-enhancing gel bra, and I was expecting to meet a woman named Sandy. Imagine my surprise when I found an old man waiting for me. He told me Sandy's father had had a heart attack, yet I still thought nothing of it.

The next step was for him to take my measurements. I had to undress to my underwear, and I was so busy freaking out that he was going to see these makeshift fake boobs with gel pads filled to the brim that it didn't occur to me to wonder why I was taking my clothes off. He had me lie on the floor, still in my underwear, my feet facing him, then asked me to lift each leg as high as I could, one at a time.

It was only when I got back into my car that I burst into tears—it suddenly hit me that none of this was right. I kept it to myself, though, as I was too embarrassed to tell my mum. I felt so stupid. Later, the police rang my home to let me know I'd encountered a known pedophile, and he was videotaping everything that happened in the room. Humiliated, I gave a statement at the police station. While this could have been the end of my career before it even began, I refused to let this person ruin my dreams. I never let this stop me from attending castings—I had no reason to be embarrassed, as I had done nothing wrong! Choose to let your bad experiences help you grow, not stop you from pursuing your dreams. I learned to listen to my gut and not let a bad first experience stop me from trying again.

Everyone wants to give you advice or opinions about how you should live your life, and not all advice is worth hearing. Find someone you love and admire, then ask for and follow their advice. The only judgment and negativity I've encountered has been from people from whom I would not even take advice—people who are more successful than me have never offered negativity. If someone offers you their advice or opinion, ask yourself, would you trade places with them? If not, why are you taking advice from them? If they are not where you want to be, and you take their advice, then you will be exactly where they are. This concept has really helped me focus on whom I should listen to and what choices I make in life.

Loving yourself also means setting aside time for self-care and personal growth. Give yourself the gift of at least thirty minutes each day for meditation or personal reflection. It's going to help you become more productive and make better decisions. Read or listen to something that inspires you every morning and spend thirty minutes meditating later in the day. If you're new to meditation, try an app, such as Calm, to get you started.

Why do you think you have to put your oxygen mask on first in an airline emergency? Because if you don't look after yourself properly, you can't look after anyone else. So often, I hear that people don't have time for themselves because of family and children. Your family doesn't need you at your worst—they need you to be on your "A game," leading as a role model. Set an example for the people who are important to you by showing them that it is just as important to care for yourself as it is to care for for others.

Hold on a second, though—let's not go too crazy with self-care! Don't coddle and protect yourself at the expense of reaching your full potential and getting out of your comfort zone. Just because something doesn't "feel" right doesn't always mean that it is not for you. It could actually be just what you need. Being in a dangerous situation is one thing—using an excuse like "I don't feel like working out; it's giving me anxiety" or "It is not 'aligning' with me" just means it's time to pull your big-girl pants on and get moving!

It's okay to be sad, ugly-cry, get it all out, and express your feelings. Then, and this is the important part, realize that you are alive, and be grateful for all the things you do have because it is more than what someone else has right now. Life happens, and it's sad sometimes, so heal from the hard times by giving back. This is the fastest way to get out of a rocky situation, depression, or difficult times.

Tasks

- Write a list of ten things that you love about yourself (your body, personality, and traits). And yes, you have to do all ten!

  1. ______________________________
  2. ______________________________
  3. ______________________________
  4. ______________________________
  5. ______________________________
  6. ______________________________
  7. ______________________________
  8. ______________________________
  9. ______________________________
  10. ______________________________

- Make a list of any negative experiences you've had recently. Give compassion to other people who might have been involved and grace to yourself. Now is the time to forgive and commit to moving on! When you experience something negative again, turn it into a positive and protect your energy.

- Schedule some "me" time in your diary. This time could involve a massage, a walk in the fresh air, or a dance party!

6. Think Bigger

It's time to level up your goals and think further outside your comfort zone! Dream bigger! Think so huge that it hurts. Most people don't want to think too big because they fear failure. Let your fear of missing out be what you fear the most. Always stretch a little more and work a little harder to reach your goals. If you fall short, you will still be so much further ahead than you imagined.

When I was fifteen, one of the projects we had to do in textiles class was to sew something over the Christmas holidays. All of my classmates were making pillowcases, blankets, or something pretty simple. You can imagine my mum's delight when I came home and told her that I, totally inexperienced at sewing, wanted to make a fifteen-layer ballet tutu with hand-embroidered details along the boned bodice!

My tutu was black and red satin and so striking, with black net layers beneath alternating black and red petal shapes in the satin material, with beading or sequins sewn around the edge. Each piece was sewn by hand and cut to perfection to make the most stunning final look. It must have taken me starting over ten times and way more time than anyone in my class, yet it was so worth it.

I was so excited to show my teacher what I had done. This teacher was known as the strictest and scariest in the whole school so if there was anyone to impress it would be her. The time had come for the grand reveal of all of our pieces we had been working on. Mine was in this huge bag, no one knew what it was, and the anticipation was killing me! My time came around. I stood up, pulled this full-on tutu out of the bag, shook it out to fluff the layers, and stood there holding it in the air. My teacher put her hands to her face, speechless and just in awe of what one of her students had done.

Think outside the box. Just because it hasn't happened yet doesn't mean it can't be done. Give something new a go. Have you had an idea out of left field that you weren't sure was going to work out? Just go for it—you will figure it out along the way by simply choosing to do it.

Find a group of friends that will stretch you. Even if you have the most incredible ideas, if the people around you don't believe in working hard and making things happen, eventually it's going to rub off on you and you will become less of who you really are. A network of people on the same page as you is essential for you to grow yourself and your business. Find people who inspire you and see how you can add value to their lives. Offer your services or assistance, and they will be there for you when you need something from them. Never go in and ask for something straightaway!

Stretch your space, too. What can you do right now with the space that you are in? My first office was in my living room in Long Beach. I bought a desk from Ikea, set it up in the living room, and got to work. When I bought my one-bedroom apartment in Huntington Beach, I decided I needed to have staff to help take my business to the next level, so I interviewed around forty people at an open-air shopping mall. So professional, right? "Hey, can you meet me outside this shop?" It worked, though, and I got two girls who started with me part-time, and we began Rebecca Louise headquarters right in my living room, with me at my desk and them working at the breakfast bar. Thanks to hard work, we eventually outgrew that apartment, and I was able to move to an office space for my entire team to grow into the next stage!

When I was fourteen, my school allowed us to choose where we would do our work experience. I always think big, so I decided I would get the hour-and-a-half train up to London each day and get my experience in another city. I wanted something more than what originally was being offered, so I found it. I may not be the smartest; I just know that with hard work and perseverance you can control some of the success that you have. At the time, I babysat for a couple; the dad worked in London at a marketing company, so I used this connection to do something different than what everyone else was doing. All I had to do was get the courage to ask if he wouldn't mind me joining him at work for a week!

Why am I sharing my personal stories and how can this help you? I want to be open and honest with you about how I got to where I am so that you are inspired to go for it yourself. As you can see, I wasn't best friends with Beyoncé; I don't have a direct number to Nike; and I didn't grow up vacationing with William and Kate. All I did was keep on going, and you can do that, too!

I am in love with the journey of working hard to help other people get to where they want to be. That chase is what keeps me going and fuels my fire. For me to help more people and have a bigger impact in the world, I needed to break out of my comfort zone. I knew I needed to be around people who were doing what I was doing and learning something new each day. Working like a hermit crab on my sofa for three years with only my dogs by my side was not allowing me to level up as much as I could! While it's easy for me to work at home, power through an amazing morning routine, and get out for a workout and to take the dogs for a walk, I know I also need to get out of my home and comfort zone to move forward. A combination of hard work and the effort to meet new people who share your passion and intention is the recipe for having ten times what you have now.

Task

- Create a vision board with everything you want to achieve in life: the family house, the destinations, the people you want to be around. Then create a bigger one, with ten times the goals and vision. Just test your mind to see where it can take you.

7. Develop Insane Belief in Yourself

There's nothing you can't do when you're focused on the mission. I believe that anything is possible for anyone when they believe they can do anything and do what needs to be done. Today I encourage you to take this concept and live by it. I mean, it's obvious, right? If you do the work you need to do to get to where you want to be, it will happen. There are no obstacles you cannot overcome when you know that it will be worth it.

I didn't own the first YouTube channel I helped to build. I appeared in most of the workout videos and put everything I had into it to help the audience get results. Then the channel simply stopped filming despite the fact it had hundreds of millions of viewers. Knowing I would have to start again from one subscriber if I was to create my own channel was a hard pill to swallow.

Even in my disappointment that the channel had stopped filming, I was still grateful that I had been part of it, because it taught me that my greatest talent in life is talking and working out at the same time! It also gave me a platform model that I could duplicate. Starting from scratch was hard work, and I didn't wake up one day feeling suddenly more motivated than I did before—with every new video I posted, every new member in our community, I felt more motivated to film and post new content. The flow of belief that I could create this on my own and provide a service for so many people who had been so adamantly asking for it all came from me simply believing I could and taking action.

When I launched my *It Takes Grit* podcast, I knew that the hardest step would be just getting it off the ground. Starting something new is no easy task, even when your business might be thriving in other areas. I knew some people only followed me for my workouts, and there was a definite fear of losing people. Yet there was something more inside me that I wanted to explore, and the platform to do it was a podcast. The first time I had opened up about many things in my life that no one knew about, it honestly was great therapy. I know it has helped many people, and I will continue to grow it to get the message out there. We're exploring big topics that talk about grit, determination, and what it takes to get to where you want to be.

And people love it! The more reviews I see, the more motivated I am to keep building this powerful platform, and that all stems from consistently taking some kind of action every day to bring in the next result.

Even when I was younger, I had belief in my abilities. "I can definitely do it myself, I don't need any help, and you can back off," I told my teachers at nursery school as they tried to help me with my laces! Thinking I was perfectly capable of completing things by myself even if it took a little longer to do it was well worth it. Yes, the teacher could have done it in two minutes rather than waiting twenty minutes for me to do it, yet that twenty minutes of me working out how to tie my shoe made it much easier in the future, when no one else was around to help me.

Don't be so quick to ask for help before you've taken five minutes to digest the question and tried to solve a problem yourself. Give learning things on your own a go—Google or YouTube it and you'll quickly build your knowledge base. I built my business and gained the skills I've needed by searching for things online. And as I was writing this book, a realization just clicked: I have not had to Google anything for this book; my thoughts have easily flowed from my heart and brain onto paper. This is because for years I believed in myself to figure it out, educate myself, and make it happen on my own. Only when I was really stuck and couldn't find the answer would I ask for help or hire someone. Looking back now, when you do it all yourself, the problems you will be faced with in the future are quickly fixed because you already know what to do. You took the time to do it on your own and figure it out. Believe in yourself—you are capable of getting the answers you need!

Even if you believe you can do anything, not everyone around you will be encouraging and supportive. I wanted to be a ballerina so badly when I was growing up. Even though I was not good enough, I would have appreciated the opportunity to give it a chance. There were two ballet exams: a standard exam and a higher-level exam you had to take in London. My teacher told me that I would have to achieve honors in my grade exam to be able to do the extra, special one that was more challenging to pass. I worked super hard, believed I could do it, and crushed the exam, coming out with honors. To my surprise, my dance teacher told me that I was in fact not allowed to do the other exam because she didn't think I would pass. Honestly, I didn't care if I passed or not. I just wanted the experience of doing it. Regardless of the way she treated me, I was determined to prove her wrong. And one day when I'm on *Dancing with the Stars*, I will have a moment to say, yes, I am good enough, and I've done it!

Even if you think you are terrible at something, go for it anyway! I wanted to be in a girl band so badly, it's probably why my fitness app has a bunch of girls in it and I have the desire for a proper tour bus for this book launch. I'm still trying to live my dream that I am in a girl band, even joining a couple of groups when I was living in London. Can I dance? Yes! Sing? Absolutely not! They would turn off my mic when we were singing, and I would just lip sync. No shame!

You can't honestly and authentically believe in other people if you don't believe in yourself. It starts with owning who you are and having positive thoughts about yourself. Go out there and own your shit and know that you can do it. Sometimes you will face people who don't believe in you, so look deep for your grit and self-assurance and don't let someone else's opinions dictate your life. The thoughts of others don't pay your bills.

Task

- Visualize who you want to be. This is such a great exercise—it will get you connected to those goals deep in your soul. Feel the fire of what you want, then use it as the fuel to push you through to reach those goals.

  Get comfortable, put on some background music that gets you fired up, and close your eyes. Spend the next five minutes imagining yourself as the person you want to be and having all the success you desire. Really elaborate the stories, play out the fantasy in your head, and visualize what it will be like when you've reached your goals and are surrounded by people who support and uplift you. After five minutes, take a deep, gentle breath in, and then exhale and slowly open your eyes. Get into the habit of doing this two or three times a week to keep that fire inside you burning.

8. Work Hard and Go the Extra Mile

Hard work beats talent. You don't need to be super-smart or know everything about a certain topic to succeed. Going the extra mile will give you an advantage over someone with natural talent who only gives 50 percent. Your 110 percent is more than their 50 percent! I was always the one at

school getting the best effort award. Sometimes it felt like a second-place trophy, and I can remember rolling my eyes, thinking, "Yes, I work the hardest, yet can I please just have the best?" Whether it was dance school, field hockey, or business, hard work can always beat talent, and always going for the goal taught me about discipline. Maybe this is why I find it so easy to work and get focused. I know how hard it can be. I trained and practiced for all those years, gave it my best, and still I wasn't considered good enough. I am sure that this just instilled in me that life isn't always easy, and things don't just come for you—you have to go after them!

By the time I was fourteen, I was great at field hockey and I was placing in dance competitions. I might have never been first, yet my hard work was paying off and I was climbing up the ranks. Sure, I was never going to be the next ballerina at the Royal Ballet; however, I proved to myself and my teachers that with hard work you will improve. It's better to work hard for something and come close to the top than not make an effort and get nowhere, simply because you didn't try. If something doesn't come naturally to you, fight for it, work hard, and soon you will have the skills to be exactly where you want to be!

Being dropped from the South of England hockey team absolutely tore me apart. I was crushed because the day I was dropped was the day I played the best game of hockey of my life. I was so mad—it just didn't make sense to me. I had extra coaching practices and one-on-one training, and I gave my all to making the cut. I went the extra mile and still it didn't happen. I didn't quit, though; I worked even harder to go back the year after for tryouts.

What I do know is that I gave it my absolute best. I did everything I needed and took all the measures possible to make the team. If you can honestly say that you are doing your best, that's all that matters. I just was not good enough; the other kids were better than me and I had to accept that. Now, if I hadn't given it everything I had, I never would have known if I could have made it. You can only do your best, so ask yourself each day if you would fire or hire yourself. Then you'll know if you have truly done all that you need to.

Going the extra mile could be making the last few reps of your workout and not stopping as the trainer counts down: "five . . . four . . . three . . . two . . . one." It might be having that extra glass of water throughout the day to maintain your hydration. Maybe you have a family event coming up and you want to make everyone something special, so they have memories of the day. If you're setting up a business and you've only told a handful of people so far, go all the way and tell everyone. Give that little bit extra of effort and push the boundaries of what you think you can do, and you will succeed. Giving your all creates momentum, and when you have momentum, all you need to do is keep your foot on the gas.

Never miss a training for an excuse. There is no reason why you can't turn up for yourself. Make the commitment to yourself that you will not skip the things you need to do to get to where you want to be. Did you know that when you miss a monthly training your business can be set back by a month and when you miss a weekly workout your results are set back a week? To think that you can slack off and still be successful is a mindset that has to change. With a structure that has already been set up for you to succeed, you just have to do the easy part and follow through and turn up.

Show yourself the discipline you have by going above and beyond to get the thing that you want, whether it's evenings, weekends, or the middle of the night. I had someone message me once asking why I'd set up a call for people to join when it was 1 AM their time. When I said, "Set your alarm and wake up," they threw back at me that as a fitness and health professional I shouldn't be encouraging people to get up in the night. Okay, sure! Because you have never been out late and gotten to bed after 1 AM or been at a sleepover where you had a midnight feast that went on for an hour? One night waking up at 1 AM is not going to kill you. Having an attitude that you can't possibly do that just means you are killing your own dreams and missing out on an opportunity.

Do one thing at a time. When it's time to work, it's time to focus on that one task. Whether it's business, exercise, or self-improvement, set aside distractions and focus on what you are doing. Finding this balance can be a constant juggle until you realize that you can only do one thing at a time successfully; multitasking is just a series of distractions. When you are spending time with family and friends, get off your phone and laptop and give them your undivided attention. Make sure you give love and care to your social life *and* your personal success. Now, if you are trying to grow a business, or maybe looking to get next-level results, it will not be a 50/50 split down the middle. In this time of growth, you'll want to spend more of your time focused on those goals. As you grow and become more, the people around you will be inspired to do more!

It makes a difference to do more in life for others. When I travel, I always try to put on a free fit camp in a park or a meet-and-greet in a hotel so that I can say hi to the people in my community. In the beginning it was just me, a music speaker, and a yoga mat, praying that at least one person would turn up. It was so daunting the first time (well, in fact, every time because I still have that "what if nobody shows" fear in the back of my mind). The fear of not doing it and missing out on meeting some of you outweighs the fear of me doing it and no one showing up, and it's always a well-attended, incredibly fun time. The extra mile is never crowded!

Tasks

- Write out the amount of time you are going to dedicate to each of your goals this week and add ten minutes to each of them. Stretch your work ethic of what you are able to do.
- Add something new into your life by learning a new skill. Write down all the ideas you have, and let's pick one to start today. Go the extra mile and do it!

9. Never Quit

There really is only one way you can fail at things: by giving up. If you give up on implementing all the ideas in this chapter, nothing will change, and you will continue to have what you always have had.

On New Year's Eve of 2017, I was excited to release the first workouts of the new year. One of the most popular New Year's resolutions is to get in shape and work out more, so I wanted to provide the perfect solution for people to achieve this. We spent time getting super creative with the workouts, all the recipes and motivation for our users to have the best experience when they opened up their app in January to kick-start their new year with a bang!

At 9 PM PST on December 31, my team members and I began receiving tons of emails and messages all across social media asking where their fitness program was, pissed off that they were paying for something that wasn't available. All our data from the app had disappeared, and as my heart sank and I felt sick, all I could think about was getting this service back up for our community who were ready to tackle those resolutions!

Dealing with people you hire who do not care about your product or your customers is challenging, and, of course, it was New Year's Eve, so we couldn't get a hold of any of the tech contractors. When the shit hits the fan, I've definitely thought about quitting, and this was one of those times. Yet that feeling of quitting disappeared in a few seconds, as serving people is always my number one priority and I couldn't let them down. The show must always go on!

Everything really is on you. When you wait for something for so long, you start to question if it will ever happen at all. The answer is that if you quit, it definitely won't happen. I believe that anyone can do anything over time as long as they don't quit. It's inevitable that if you never give up and stick to it, something will come of it.

Embrace the days when you're struggling. Lean into those difficult days—they're a sign you're almost ready for the next level of your life.

Appreciate these times of growth and use your experience in the future. Flip your mindset and get excited when things start to become a challenge; it only means you are making the things that happened before seem too easy. The universe is leveling up its game to take you to the next phase of your life so all you get to do is rise up!

Looking back, I can't believe how many times I've experience rejection for castings and job opportunities. My ratio was probably 90 percent "no" to 10 percent "yes." I was so eager to make it happen, knowing that if I kept showing up, I would eventually get *something*. Securing a job was the best feeling ever—making the cut or being part of something new was so exciting after facing rejection and endlessly preparing myself to hear "no." And even though there were auditions where I was completely rubbish, stood out like a sore thumb, and was not even close to being selected, I was gaining experience and trying to live out my dreams rather than be miserable and mope on the sofa.

If I had hidden away and not been around the buzz, I don't feel like my spark would have stayed alive. When you quit going to the gym, you stop being around healthy people working out. You remove yourself from your goal; when you do that, it's out of sight, out of mind. The dream dies and slips away from you. If you're thinking about quitting, find that fire and keep on doing the things that will help you stay on track. When I was getting more rejections than jobs, I knew that backing off would put me farther away from my goals.

Come back to your "why" when you feel like giving up. Is giving up your big hopes and dreams ever worth it? Absolutely not! Don't quit for anything. How can you face yourself in the mirror knowing that the only reason you didn't achieve what you set out to was because you quit—not because you weren't good enough, didn't know enough, or weren't capable, but simply because you quit? And if you quit on something in the past, it's not too late, because you are still here! Start again and you'll see that you didn't quit; you just took a break.

Expect rejection! Then anything other than that is just a bonus when it does happen for you. As long as you have given your best, done the work, and shown up, you can't expect to be picked every time or have results as soon as you would like. Really prepare yourself for things to go wrong and know that you are not going to quit when something goes south—you are just going to work to get through it.

Tasks

- Make a list of the things that will make you feel like you want to quit at your journey.

  Example: I think I'm not good enough; I don't think I have the time; It is too hard right now.

  Then when you want to quit, look at this list and ask yourself:

  1. Is it worth quitting for any one of these things?
  2. Is it worth losing your dream because of any one of these?

- Create a poster that says "NEVER GIVE UP—JUST LEVEL UP." Put it in your house where you can see it daily. We all need a visual reminder to grab our attention and keep us focused. Make it pretty, something you enjoy looking at, and of course place it where you can frequently see it.

10. Take Action!

Just get started, and give yourself permission to be messy! You are going to be rubbish at the beginning, you will not know what to do, and you will have to clean it up as you go. You do not have to be great to start; you have to start to be great.

Don't focus on perfection. You will never be 100 percent ready, so all you are doing by delaying is making sure that nothing will ever change. No one expects you to have it all figured out on day one. Even now I am always learning new things and still don't have it all figured out—we never will!

I love drawing things out and being creative. Once you've come up with an idea, you'll probably run into some roadblocks. When that happens, push them to one side, and follow through with your idea by getting it in front of someone who can help you bring it to life. When I created my app, I started by drawing it on paper—what was going to link to what and how it was all going to function. Once this was done (and it was far from perfect), I got in touch with some developers who could bring this vision of mine to life.

With no investor or trust fund, I quickly found that my roadblock was that I was just scraping by with a small budget. Technology isn't cheap, and if you want something done well, the last thing you want is to cut corners. It was incredibly demotivating for me to find that everyone I met with was out of my price range, and even if I'd sold my house, I didn't have the capital. I was 100 percent sold on my idea and knew that it would be great. Without half a million dollars to make it happen, I just had to keep looking for someone new to app development or outsource it to another country.

The more action you take, the more you will get motivated. With every meeting I had with developers, the more I learned, and the closer I got to that pot of gold. It was almost like I was on a treasure hunt, finding clues along the way about how to get to the final destination.

My motivation comes from constantly casting a big vision for myself, looking forward into the future, and dreaming about how it will feel when it happens. Get fired up thinking about what will happen to you in the future as you implement these steps. You are either growing or dying, and without a strong vision for yourself, you are dying. It's your vision—what you want is all right there in your heart and it's totally possible for you to achieve. Say it out loud, write it down, close your eyes, and visualize yourself living out your dreams.

Motivation comes from action. Start by doing the action and you will find the motivation. Switch your mindset here on what you think is going to come first. No one ever got motivated by sitting around wishing something was going to happen. Those excited endorphins start to come in after you have just done a little bit and seen the smallest of results. Your brain tells you that if you do more, you are going to get more, which will keep you motivated and on track for your goals.

When I was younger, I wanted so badly to go to private school, yet my parents didn't have enough money to send me. Instead of accepting that I couldn't go, I applied for scholarships to make it possible. I wasn't giving up just because my situation at the time didn't allow it. I went to meet the headmaster and gave him every reason why I should get this scholarship. I told him that I would be a great student, he could rely on me, and that I would add value to the school. I got the scholarship and was able to go to the school I desired. Unfortunately, on my first day, a girl who bullied me at dance class told everyone to bully me before leaving the school herself. So, I was at my dream school, working in the library most lunch times by myself, feeling scared to go and eat with everyone else. I became depressed and my weight dropped down to 86 pounds. I decided to stick it out and focus on my schoolwork, and I walked away from that school with four A levels—three As and a B. Keep going, and do it for yourself even when your environment is not the most supportive.

Learn the skills you need to gain confidence. When you know how to do something well, you are much more likely to keep at it. The only way you get good at something is by doing it over and over again. A lack of confidence is 100-percent curable! If you know you are not confident in something, the best way to feel more in control is by educating yourself or doing more of what you want to achieve. There is no easier way to get better at something than by simply doing it. Break the pattern and take action, and you will soon find yourself with all of the confidence and motivation you need to succeed.

My high school sports teams were crap, and no one wanted to be part of them. I would run around in the morning, begging people to play just so we had enough players to turn up. I would spend my lunch breaks calling other schools and trying to schedule games because I didn't feel enough was being done by our teachers to organize games. I wanted to play, and I took action. And I never gave up—I knew with enough shameless begging and probably bribery I could get my classmates to stand on that field. In retrospect, it didn't help that our hockey shirts looked like clown outfits!

Get laser-focused. Stay in your lane, stay the course, and remain a student always. When you are distracted, you do less work and therefore your results and motivation suffer. Stay on the journey and be laser-focused about everything that you are doing. When things don't go quite to plan or we don't get the results as soon as we think we should, we often move away from the path that was created for us to be successful. Don't deviate from that road map; you will lose momentum and motivation. Stick to the path and jump over the barrels that come your way, and you will be on a guaranteed path to success.

Tasks

- Map out your ninety-day plan to kickstart your road to results, and write down three things you need to do each day to help you achieve your goals. We can make big lists of everything we need to do and totally overwhelm ourselves, not even lasting a week. Committing to those three things and then actually doing them will give you a sense of accomplishment that will motivate you to continue. Don't expect to see results until you have done something for ninety days. Consider any results you achieve before that a bonus!

- Map out your six-month, one-year, three-year, five-year, and ten-year plans using all the tools you've learned so far. Now multiply those goals by ten! Is there something in your five-year plan that you can accomplish in six months? Push yourself and take action today.

PART II

FOOD AND FITNESS

5

Your Balanced Diet

What you put into your body is so important! I always say that abs are made in the kitchen, and I'll say it again: Of how you look and feel, 80 percent is due to what you eat, 20 percent is fitness, and 100 percent is your mindset! Learning to balance your diet is essential to your success. Without proper nutrition, your body won't be able to perform at its best, so it's crucial to understand how to make healthy, tasty meals that are packed with nutrients.

A poor diet opens the door to disease, fatigue, infections, and unhealthy skin. When I was younger and struggling with an eating disorder, I had terrible acne, lack of energy, and mood swings. Once I reevaluated my diet and figured out how to properly balance my plate, I was able to regain control over my skin, my weight, *and* my life.

A balanced diet includes the right nutrients, as well as knowing how much food you need to eat to stay healthy and active. In this chapter, we will cover everything you need to know about portion control, meal planning and preparation, hydration, and supplements.

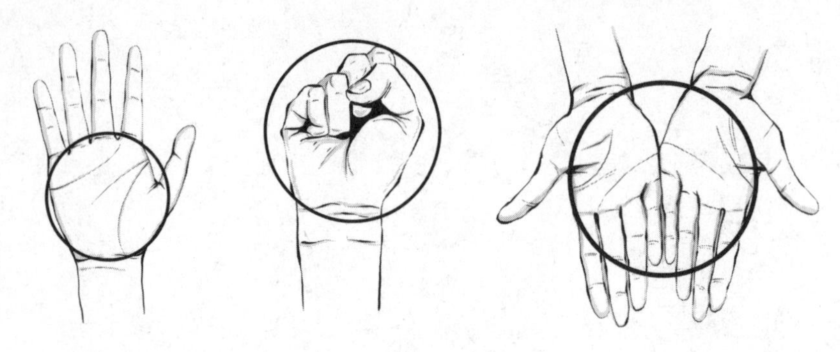

Don't have a kitchen scale to measure your food portions? No problem! Use your hands as a guide. You can do this anywhere!

Portion Control

The perfect plate contains a balance of protein, whole-grain carbohydrates, lots of fresh vegetables, plus healthy fats. When planning your meal, include a palm-size portion of protein, a fist-size portion of healthy whole grains, and enough fresh veggies to fill your cupped hands (or half of your plate). Add a small amount of olive oil, avocado, nuts, or other heathy fats, and dig in!

Food Groups

A healthy diet includes a balance of carbohydrates, protein, and fats. Choosing these foods in the right proportions is the key. Each day, you should aim for about 40 percent carbohydrates, 30 percent protein, and 30 percent fat. While you may find that some meals have more carbs, fat, or protein than others, at the end of the day, it should all balance out. If you're new to meal planning, don't worry! You'll find healthy recipes with these guidelines in mind in Chapter 11, as well as a detailed meal plan for each day of the challenge.

Carbohydrates: 40 Percent of Your Diet

There are two types of carbohydrates: complex and simple. Complex carbs are whole foods that contain vitamins, minerals, and antioxidants, plus a healthy dose of fiber. Oatmeal, brown rice, quinoa, potatoes, beans, peas, and lentils are examples of foods rich in complex carbohydrates. Complex carbohydrates break down slowly, providing you with sustained energy and level blood sugar throughout the day.

Simple carbohydrates are found in processed foods like white bread, white rice, and baked goods. Soda, candy, and sweeteners such as sugar, maple syrup, and honey are also simple carbs. These easily digested carbohydrates are rapidly absorbed, causing a spike in blood sugar and a quick boost in energy while delivering fewer nutrients. Most foods contain carbohydrates, including fruits, vegetables, and some dairy products, but because they contain fiber and essential nutrients, they should be consumed daily.

Fiber is an essential part of your diet—it regulates blood sugar, prevents heart disease, and keeps you "regular." Enjoy a fiber-rich diet of greens, apples, oats, peas, potatoes, carrots, barley, and green beans. If you know that you need to take a trip to the loo, and need a little help, then eat some fiber to help pass things along. There are two types of fiber, and you need both of them. Soluble fiber, found in foods like beans, oats, fruits, peas, and potatoes, attracts water and slows digestion, while insoluble fiber, found in whole grains, seeds, and the skins of fruits and veggies, adds bulk and helps food move through your system efficiently. Depending on your age and gender, you'll want to consume between 21 and 38 grams of fiber each day.

Complex Versus Simple Carbs

Complex carbs are your "good carbs." They nourish you and give you energy.

- Brown rice
- Legumes: beans, lentils, green peas, and chickpeas
- Barley
- Quinoa
- Oatmeal
- Green vegetables
- Sweet potatoes
- Carrots
- Apples
- Citrus fruits
- Winter squash
- 100 percent whole wheat breads and pasta
- Farro

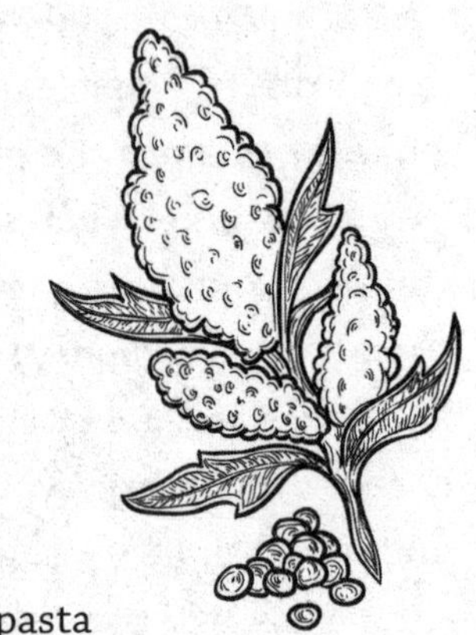

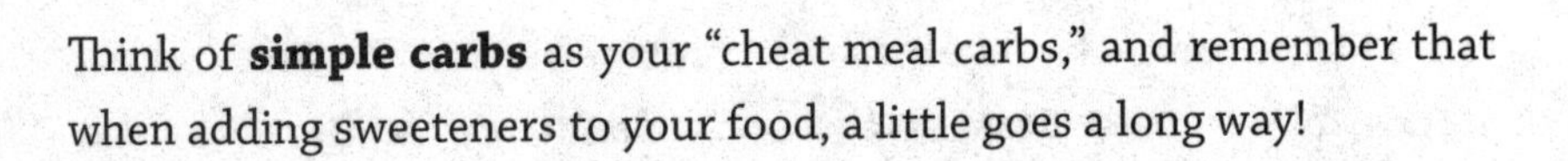

Think of **simple carbs** as your "cheat meal carbs," and remember that when adding sweeteners to your food, a little goes a long way!

- Fair food: funnel cakes, corn dogs, and fried cookies
- Ice cream
- Cookies
- Candy
- Sweetened coffee shop drinks
- Soda
- Chips
- Fast food
- Sugar: white/brown sugar, honey, raw sugar, coconut sugar, maple syrup
- Sweetened breakfast cereal
- Fruit juice

Best Fruits and Vegetables to Eat

Choose a rainbow of vegetables every day—eating your colors ensures that you're getting a wide variety of macro- and micronutrients in your diet. Fill half of your plate with vegetables at each meal, aiming for four to five servings of fresh veggies every day.

Broccoli and kale. Broccoli is packed with nutrients, including a healthy dose of fiber, vitamins C and K, iron, and potassium, and it contains more protein than most other veggies. Loaded with vitamins and minerals, kale has long been considered a "superfood." It provides more vitamin C than an orange per serving, along with rich amounts of fiber and vitamin A.

Blueberries, blackberries, and raspberries. Berries are essential to a healthy diet—they contain more antioxidants and less sugar than other fruits, and they're full of fiber, too. Studies have shown that eating berries protects you from heart disease, stroke, diabetes, and cognitive decline.

Tomatoes. Tomatoes are rich in vitamin C and fiber, as well as the antioxidant lycopene, which protects against heart disease and certain cancers.

Avocados. Avocados are full of fiber, the antioxidant vitamin E, and healthy unsaturated fats. Having enough fat in your diet is essential to help your body absorb fat-soluble nutrients such as vitamins E, D, and K. Avocados also inhibit the production of inflammatory chemicals in your body.

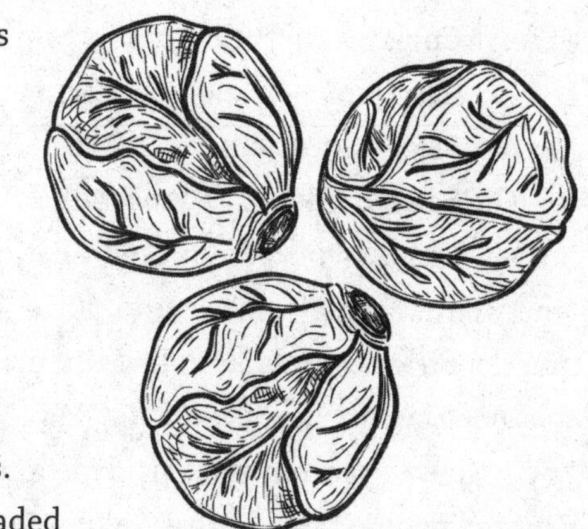

Brussels sprouts. These tiny cabbage-like vegetables are a great source of B vitamins. Brussels sprouts are also loaded with fiber and vitamins A, C, and K. A ½ cup serving of Brussels sprouts is only 25 calories, so enjoy them steamed, roasted, or raw in a salad.

Leafy greens. Leafy greens such as spinach, Swiss chard, arugula, lettuces, and mustard greens are packed with vitamins and minerals. Eating several servings of greens a day protects against heart disease and cognitive decline and promotes healthy digestion and clear skin. Enjoy your greens in soups, salads, or pasta dishes, or simply steamed as a side with a drizzle of olive oil and lemon.

Protein: 30 Percent of Your Diet

Protein is an essential part of your diet. It is a basic building block of your body as all muscle tissue contains protein. To maintain the muscle mass of a sedentary adult you will want to consume .4 grams of protein per pound of body weight (.88 grams of protein per kilogram). For active adults, this number increases, as you'll need to eat more protein to maintain what you burn off during exercise. For a strength-focused fitness plan, aim for .5 to .8 grams of protein per pound of body weight (1.2 to 1.7 grams per kilogram), while endurance athletes should aim for .5 to .6 grams per pound (1.2 to 1.5 grams per kilogram).

For a balanced diet, no more than 35 percent of your daily caloric intake should come from protein. Eating excess protein is wasteful, as your body can only use around 30 to 40 grams at a time for building muscle mass. When you follow the meal and snack plan in Part III of this book, you'll be eating your daily protein number of about 90 to 160 grams of protein per day, depending on your height, weight, gender, and goals. If you're already fit and looking to gain weight and add muscle, you can increase these numbers—try increasing your daily protein intake by about 10 to 15 grams per day while increasing your weights during your workouts for two weeks and see how your body adapts.

Before you ask, nope—you are not going to bulk up by meeting your daily requirements for protein intake and physical activity, and no, a high-protein diet is not healthier. You need to eat a balance of protein, carbs, and fat for a healthy body. To bulk up, you'd have to eat massive amounts of food and lift hundreds of pounds of weight consistently for years. You will not wake up one morning looking like the Incredible Hulk! Don't be afraid to eat your daily recommended amount and pick up some heavier weights!

Protein Sources

Animal Proteins

Chicken and turkey. Poultry provides lower-fat, healthy protein that's easy to cook and have on hand for meal prep. Look for skinless, boneless breasts or thighs, lean ground turkey, or sliced lower-sodium turkey and chicken from the deli department.

Red meat. Lean red meats can be an excellent source of protein; however, there are health risks to excessive intake of red meat, so consider this a treat meal and not a daily choice. Choose grass-fed whenever possible, and stick to the lower-fat cuts of beef, pork, or lamb.

Fish. As a pescatarian, I get lots of my protein from fish and seafood. Choose a variety of oily, omega 3–rich fish like wild salmon or tuna, flaky white fish like cod or halibut, and mineral-rich shellfish such as shrimp or clams.

Vegetarian Proteins

Tofu, tempeh, and edamame. Choose organic soy products whenever possible. Edamame are simply steamed soybeans in their pods. They're available in the freezer department, and they're one of nature's perfectly balanced foods—a ½ cup serving is 100 calories and contains a near-perfect mix of 38 percent carbs, 34 percent protein, and 28 percent fat. Tofu and tempeh are versatile foods that provide healthy protein for your plant-based meals. Try tofu in a breakfast scramble (Tofu Veggie Scramble on page 243) or a healthy salad (Sweet Tofu and Cauliflower Salad on page 258), or use sliced or crumbled tempeh or tofu in place of meat in your favorite recipe.

Vegetables. All vegetables contain protein, so eating a wide variety will help you to reach your daily protein goals. Veggies such as broccoli, avocado, Brussels sprouts, potatoes, and asparagus are packed with protein, plus healthy fiber and nutrients.

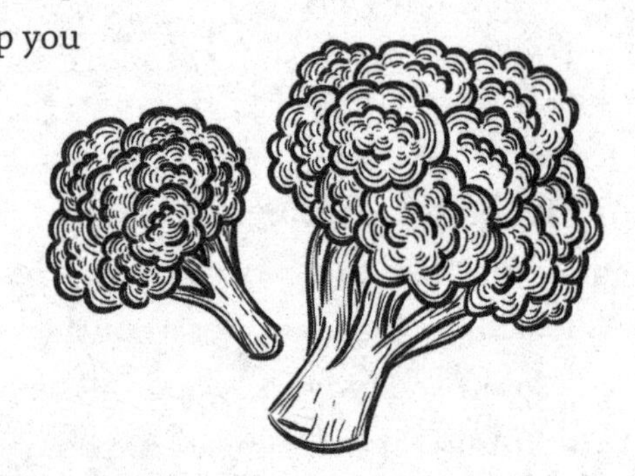

Beans and legumes. Green peas, lentils, chickpeas, mung beans, black beans, pinto beans . . . the list goes on! Beans and legumes are a fantastic source of protein, and they're full of fiber and healthy carbs, which keep you full, regulate your blood sugar, and keep that healthy digestion moving along.

Protein powder. Protein powders and shakes containing soy, whey, rice, or pea protein are a great choice for your breakfast shake, protein pancakes, or a post-workout shake—the next section goes in depth on the different varieties and when I use them.

Is Soy an Estrogen?

Soy gets a bad rap: "It's full of estrogen!" "Your sons will have man boobs!" While we all have estrogen in our bodies that comes from fat in our bloodstream, especially after age fifty, it's not soy that causes these issues. Soy contains antioxidant soy isoflavones (genistein and daidzein). According to David Heber, MD, PhD, and professor emeritus/founder of the UCLA Center for Human Nutrition, soy isoflavones bind only 1/1000 as much as estradiol (the strongest estrogen found in your bloodstream), and these isoflavones actually block the binding of estrogens to protein. Your bones, heart, and brain contain receptors that bind these isoflavones, estrogens, and other phytonutrients called phytoestrogens. Soy consumption has been linked to reduced incidences of breast cancer, osteoporosis, and menopause symptoms. If you've had cancer, it's worth talking to your doctor about how much soy is right for you, otherwise feel free to enjoy soy protein, as well as soy foods, such as edamame, tofu, and tempeh, as part of your healthy diet.

Protein Powders and Shakes

There are many options for choosing a protein powder for making healthy shakes.

Soy protein. Soy protein is made from soybeans and is one of the few plant-based protein powders that contain all nine essential amino acids, which are the building blocks of protein that our body cannot produce on its own. It is generally made after the soybeans have been hulled, dried, and then turned into soy flour.

Soy protein is a great choice for meal replacement shakes and breakfast smoothies.

Whey protein. Whey is one of the most popular protein powders on the market today; I use it for my post-workout shake. It is the liquid byproduct of cheese production, and it can also be made from milk. Whey is quickly absorbed by the body and is relatively cheap in comparison to other types of protein powders. There are different types of whey protein available, so when you are looking for one to buy, it is a good idea to know what each of them are.

Whey protein concentrate (WPC) is generally the cheapest type of whey protein because it has the lowest amount of protein per 100 grams when compared to the other two. That being said, it still has quite a high percentage of protein, which can vary from about 60 to 90 percent. The rest is typically made up of fat, carbohydrates (lactose), and other peptides.

Whey protein isolate (WPI) has a protein content of about 90 to 95 percent, with minimal lactose and fat. My preferred choice of whey protein, it is one of the most popular forms of protein.

Whey protein hydrolysate (WPH) is the type of whey with the highest amount of protein per 100 grams at 99 percent. This type of protein is usually the most expensive and can have a stronger flavor, which may make it harder to mask with other ingredients.

Pea protein. This is a popular protein choice for both vegetarians and vegans. Made from yellow split peas, pea protein generally doesn't have many additives or artificial ingredients, so it's one of the few proteins that is as close to the whole food source as possible. It is also free from soy, gluten, and lactose, making it a good choice if you have food allergies. Your body can absorb pea protein quite easily, and it has a high protein content for a plant-based protein, making it a great choice if you prefer to avoid animal products.

Rice protein. As its name suggests, rice protein comes from rice, commonly brown rice. While it does contain protein, the fact that rice is a grain means that it has a higher carbohydrate content in comparison to other protein powders. However, it is certainly another suitable choice for vegetarians or vegans.

For a delicious breakfast shake, try my Reboot Spinach and Almond Butter Smoothie (page 235) with your favorite protein powder. For a healthy post-workout shake choose one that has whey protein, BCAAs (branch chain amino acids), and L-glutamines that you just mix with water. There is no need to add bananas, yogurt, or anything else—keep it clean and simple! Read your nutrition labels and choose what's best for you. Unlike whey and soy, both pea and rice proteins do not contain all nine essential amino acids. If you are planning on using either of these as protein supplements, you may need to incorporate other foods to make sure that you are meeting your body's protein needs. While protein powders are a convenient way to get your daily protein, they should not be used to completely replace protein foods, rather as part of a healthy, varied diet consisting of whole foods.

Fats: Up to 30 Percent of Your Diet

You definitely need those good fats! Your body cannot naturally produce fatty acid, so it needs to come from the food you eat. Without fat, you wouldn't have the energy you need to get through your day. Fats also provide essential nutrients, protect your bones, and promote healthy skin and digestion. Without it, you're nothing but (unhealthy) skin and bones! Aim to get about 30 percent of your calories from fat. Stay away from large amounts of trans fats, which are present in processed foods such as cakes, cookies, and frozen convenience foods. Choose whole foods like avocados and nuts, or unprocessed oils like olive or coconut, and enjoy dairy fats like butter and cheese in moderation. Consider processed foods and baked goods an occasional "cheat" rather than something you regularly enjoy.

Healthy Fats Versus "Bad" Fats

Healthy fats should be in the foods you eat on a daily basis.

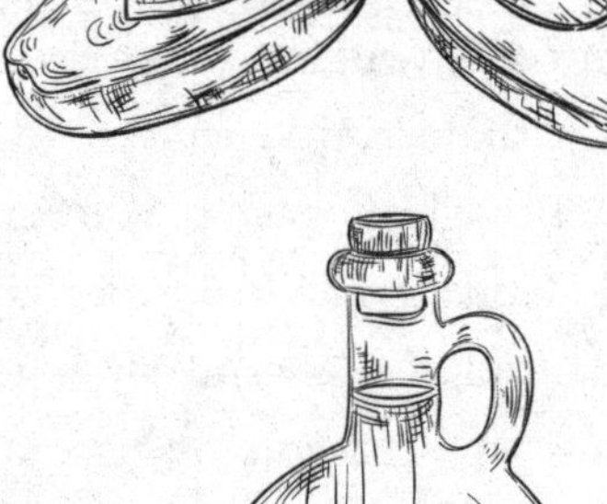

- Avocado
- Extra-virgin olive oil
- Flax meal and seeds
- Coconut oil
- Butter (in moderation)
- Cheese (in moderation)
- Eggs
- Fatty fish (such as salmon)
- Nuts
- Dark chocolate (in moderation)

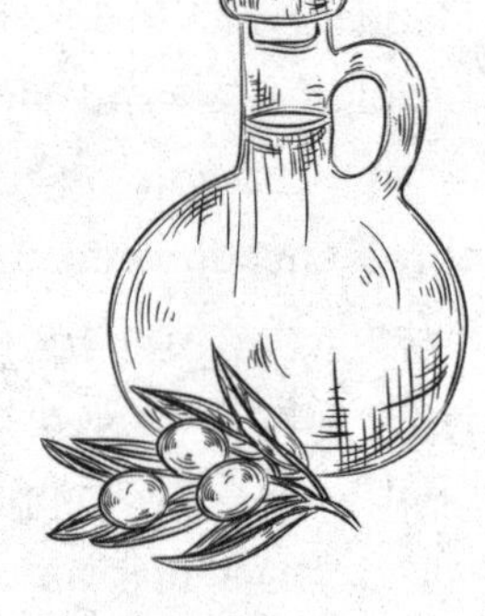

"Bad" fats are in those unhealthy foods you should only eat every once in a while.

- Margarine
- Doughnuts
- Processed meats
- Canola oil
- Cookies
- French fries
- Frozen pizzas and meals
- Fried fish
- Creamers and coffee shop drinks
- Takeout and fast food

Water

Drinking plenty of water is essential for good health. I drink about 3 liters per day. I recommend 2.7 liters for women and 3.7 liters for men. When you are working out, it's necessary to drink more water to replenish what you have lost. It's also a good idea to drink water with electrolytes to get the water quickly back to the muscles so you can continue with a good workout.

Vitamins and Minerals

Vitamins and minerals help your body to develop and function at an optimal level. It doesn't have to be difficult—if you're eating a healthy and balanced diet, with colorful meals and good supplements, then you will be getting all you need.

There are two different types of vitamins: water-soluble and fat-soluble. There are thirteen essential vitamins: A, B, C, D, E, K, B1, B2, B3, B6, B7, B9, and B12. Vitamins A, D, E, and K are fat-soluble, so if you consume too much, they are stored in your liver, while the others are water-soluble—your body releases any excess in your urine. Each vitamin plays an important role in protecting your health and combating a variety of diseases. Vitamin-rich foods include all whole foods, such as fruits like watermelon, berries, avocados, and citrus; meats such as fish, poultry, and beef; legumes; dairy products; vegetables; soy products; and whole grains.

Minerals, which are as necessary as vitamins, are elements that we absorb directly or indirectly from the environment or from the animal that ate them. Important dietary minerals include calcium, chloride, magnesium, potassium, sodium, iron, chromium, copper, fluoride, iodine, and zinc.

If you eat a variety of colors, you will live a colorful life. Phytonutrients are present in bright and vibrant fruits and veggies. They boost your health and well-being and play a role in protecting your immune system. To get your phytonutrients in, think about eating the rainbow. Make sure your plate is colorful with green, red, and yellow peppers, bright red tomatoes, sweet potatoes, mangos, berries, and dark leafy greens like kale or spinach.

Supplements are a great way to complement your nutrition plan and fill in the gaps where needed. Supplements should not replace food—rather, combine them with whole foods throughout the day. A protein-rich meal replacement shake that includes carbohydrates, good fats, and vitamins and minerals is a great way to start your day and can help boost your metabolism first thing in the morning. Other supplements I recommend throughout the day include a post-workout shake and a multivitamin tablet to provide your body with the recommended daily intake of micronutrients. To ensure your body is also receiving healthy fats to improve brain and heart health, consider adding an omega 3 supplement as well.

Choosing organic foods will help ensure that you don't ingest unwanted pesticides and chemicals that can be toxic and harmful to your body. Organic foods may have higher nutritional value and better flavor than conventionally grown, as the absence of pesticides and fertilizers may boost plants' production of phytonutrients. Organic farming also helps protect the environment by reducing pollution and conserving water. Choose organic whenever your budget allows.

Simple Meal Plan

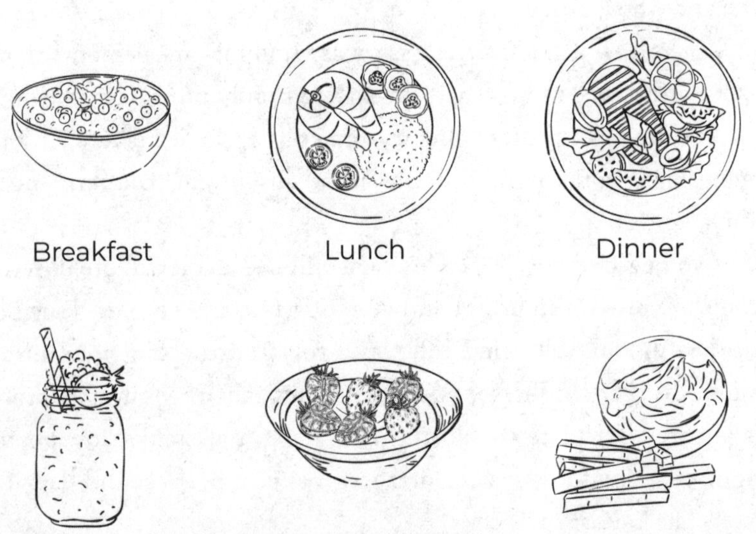

Preparing a Healthy Meal

Choose healthy carbs. Choose fiber-rich complex carbs over simple carbs. Complex carbs (such as whole grains or starchy vegetables) are really good for you, while simple carbs (such as refined grains) will turn to sugar in your body, which then turns to fat.

Roast your vegetables. Use just a touch of olive oil, salt, and pepper to add flavor.

Lightly dress your salad. Instead of thick, heavy, calorie-dense dressings, keep it simple with a little bit of salt and pepper and a small amount of oil and vinegar or fresh lemon juice.

Grill your protein. Stick to about 20 to 30 grams of grilled, broiled, or baked protein. Never deep-fry.

Add some flavor. Sometimes a little salt and freshly ground pepper are all you need, or a simple squeeze of lemon. Need a little something more? Make healthy sauces with puréed veggies, curry paste, and coconut milk, or canned plum tomatoes with lots of fresh veggies. Or try using fresh herbs and dried spices to add flavor to your meals.

Snacks

Let's talk about snacks! It's easy to pick up a bag of chips or order that side of truffle fries (my weakness) when you're in a snacking mood. Before you give in to your cravings, ask yourself if it's really worth it. Now, I'm not saying that you're not allowed to splurge every now and then; just be mindful of healthier snack alternatives that will ultimately leave you feeling more satisfied in the long run and sustain your energy. Some people believe that eating healthy means *zero* snacks; that couldn't be more wrong! I eat at least three snacks (mid-morning, afternoon, and evening), and I very rarely have a rumbling stomach. As long as you are working out regularly, eating three healthy meals and three healthy snacks will not contribute to weight gain.

Read your labels and mind your protein! Women should keep snacks to around 10 to 15 grams of protein, while men should aim for 15 to 20 grams. Be sure that your protein count is higher than fat or carbs. For snacking inspiration and ideas, turn to page 140.

Foods to Avoid

Not all foods are created equal, and there are some that have no place in a healthy diet. Avoid these foods in your daily diet, and if you must have an occasional "cheat meal," do so in moderation and then get right back on your healthy eating plan!

Soda is high in sugar and sodium. It dehydrates you and leads to gum disease, weight gain, and metabolic issues.

Fried foods are high in calories and trans fats that clog arteries and increase cholesterol.

White foods (such as pasta, rice, and white bread) are high in simple sugars that increase your blood sugar and insulin, leading to overeating.

Candy and chocolate are low in nutrients and can cause insulin resistance, heart disease, and diabetes.

Tasks

- Write down what you ate and drank over the last three days. Using a different color, add in any missing meals or snacks so you can see where you can improve. With another color, mark where you could have chosen a healthier alternative.

- Now let's take one of your meals that you've cooked in the last three days and see what you can change to make it a healthier version. Let's go ahead and make it! Don't look at the recipes in this book for inspiration right now; I want to teach you how you can use these tools to make any meal healthy so in the future you'll always be able to make food that tastes good and is good for you, too!

- It's time to clear out: Go through your pantry and fridge and get rid of soda, unhealthy frozen meals, candy, cakes, and cookies. Simply not having them there is the first step to not eating them. Donate the unopened food instead of throwing it away.

6

Healthy Food Habits

Now that you've learned the basics of healthy meal planning and nutrition, you probably feel like you have more questions than answers! Reviewing your food choices may make you wonder about healthy alternatives to the foods you don't want to give up. And what about stress eating, managing cravings and PMS, and restaurant meals? You're probably thinking, "Rebecca, I need my dinners out and a glass of wine!" Don't panic, because I'm going to help you to find the balance that will keep you happy and healthy.

Small changes, swaps, and alternatives can make all the difference to your results and health. I don't recommend that you make all of these changes in one go—if this list seems overwhelming, start with a few swaps and keep adding more each week. Tell yourself, "Okay, for the next month I am going to take out soda and replace it with water." Just for one month! Then after that see how your body feels, and when you do have soda again be aware of the reaction you might have. It's like alcohol—I love a glass of prosecco, yet if I have it every day the effect of the buzz wears off, and I'm just drinking poison. A few times each year,

I'll skip alcohol for a couple of months, and when I do treat myself to a glass, I'm giggling a few sips in. Well, that's me anyway. It shows me that when I consume too much booze, my body simply gets used to it. Ever been to a music festival and, by the third day, you are four drinks in and you still can't feel anything? Yeah, that's dangerous!

You only begin to notice how food and drinks make you feel when you haven't had them for a while. I eat pretty clean, and when I do eat fast food, I feel gross, like I'm exploding from the waist down! Start eliminating the foods that aren't good for you and see how much lighter you feel, and how your energy levels soar!

Alternative Food Choices

Instead of	**Try**
Starchy white potato	Sweet potato
Sugary milk chocolate	Dark chocolate
Candy	Dried fruits
Potato chips	Kale chips
French fries	Baked veggie fries
White pasta and noodles	Zucchini noodles
Milkshakes	Fruit smoothies
Soda	Water
Ice cream	Frozen yogurt
Chocolate pudding	Chia seed pudding
Mashed potatoes	Mashed cauliflower
Candy bar	Protein bar
Salty tortilla chips	Plantain chips with salsa
Jam	Smashed avocado
Mayo	Hummus
White rice	Quinoa or brown rice
Sour cream	Unsweetened Greek yogurt

Instead of	Try
Croutons	Almonds
Iceberg lettuce	Romaine lettuce
Creamy salad dressings	Oil and vinegar
Peanut butter	Almond butter
Whole milk	Unsweetened almond milk
Sugary fruit juices	Fruit-infused water
Popsicles	Frozen grapes
Sugary cereal	Oatmeal

Stress Eating

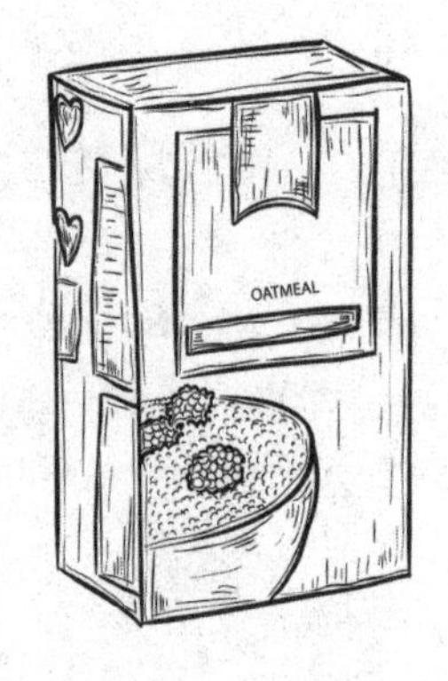

I can demolish chocolate—if it's in my house it will not last for more than a night. I have to stop myself from buying it or I will binge-eat it all. There are times when I feel sad and I want to eat all the bad foods. When those feelings strike, I get it out of my system for one evening only; when the new day starts, I am back to my routine.

I have learned balance in my life, so sometimes I'll go out for a three-course dinner, yet the next day I'm back to eating clean and getting in a hard workout. This is how I have been able to maintain my physique and still live my life: 80 percent of me is clean eating and daily workouts, and 20 percent is prosecco and chocolate!

Tips to Manage Stress Eating

Start a food journal.

This practice doesn't have to be all about diet. Your notebook can be a reflection of your day in general: what you did, how you felt, and what you ate. You'll be able to identify what triggers food cravings and sensations of hunger (even when your body may already be satisfied). A journal is a good way to stay accountable and make associations between stress and your eating habits.

Work out.

Get those endorphins flying, your body moving, and the energy flowing by exercising. Exercise can take your mind off the events of the day, distract you from eating, and also burn calories. After your workout, you can go grab your recovery shake!

Just wait.

What's the worst thing that could happen if you don't follow through with the urge to eat? Rather than immediately giving in, drink some water and find an activity to do that will delay your cravings and binges. You might find that an impulse will simply pass after a bit of time has gone by, and you'll feel better without being weighed down by unnecessary foods.

Be kind to yourself.

Eating as a response to stress is a pretty good indicator that whatever the issue might be, it's not being addressed or resolved. Channel negative or stressful thoughts into something creative, productive, or helpful for others. Give yourself time to unlearn habits like stress eating, and don't be too hard on yourself if it doesn't come naturally at first. Practice and persistence is what really counts.

Nutrition Q&A

Once you dive into really analyzing your diet and swapping bad foods and habits for good ones, it's time to go the extra mile. Let's look at your next steps and answer your burning questions about food!

Can I drink alcohol?

It depends on the kind of results that you want and by when. Although I do drink very occasionally, I notice a huge change in my results when I cut out alcohol. I am leaner and stronger and my mind is clear—obviously! Booze is a poison that will slow down your metabolism, and let's not even talk about trying to work out with a hangover! If you choose to drink alcohol, cut down your consumption and avoid sugary cocktails that will give you a pounding headache in the morning. The leanest drink you can have is straight tequila on ice. The choice is yours: How badly do you want to see those results?

If I miss a snack, should I have it later with my meal?

We all have days when we miss meals and snacks. This is one thing I wouldn't be doubling up on. Your body can only digest a certain amount of protein at once, so if you're shoveling more in, you're doing more harm than good. Simply go to the next meal or snack on your plan.

What should I eat after a workout?

I choose to have a post-workout recovery shake because it is quick and easy and has all the essential items in there to repair and recover at an optimal level.

When you put a flower in the sun, it starts to grow, yet if you don't feed it water it will die. It needs both elements to keep it alive. The same goes for your body—when you work out, you are taxing and tearing your muscles during exercise, breaking your fibers down. The most important part of exercise is what you eat after, so you'll want to choose a shake or snack that promotes repair.

You can choose a protein-rich snack after you work out if you don't want to have a shake. Just make sure that if it's something you have to cook you prep it beforehand, so you can eat within thirty minutes of completing your workout.

What should I eat before a workout and how long before?

I recommend eating a snack thirty to forty-five minutes before your workout. You need energy for your workout, which means eating protein and complex carbs. For snack ideas, turn to page 140.

How do I control cravings?

Eat regularly and make sure each meal and snack contains protein to keep you feeling full. Having a healthy breakfast that includes protein, complex carbs, and good fats will also maintain your blood sugar level, which can control those feelings of needing something sugary or salty. Eat regular meals and snacks—don't let yourself get to a point of starvation, because this is when you'll grab whatever food you see, rather than making a decision based on your health and goals. We all have cravings, and it's okay to have that treat, in moderation. This life is to be enjoyed, so don't beat yourself up if you have a piece of cake or a bag of chips. One bad meal is not going to spoil your results, just like one healthy meal isn't going to get you abs!

Are there certain foods I should avoid at certain times of the day?

I recommend eating the majority of your carbohydrates for breakfast and pre- and post-workout because this is what will give you the energy you need for the day. If you are going to have a treat like chocolate or sweets, have it during the day. Avoid these foods just before you go to bed, because during sleep your body cannot as easily burn off the sugar calories.

What about fasting?

I understand fasting works for many people. I have found that I am looking for a lifestyle that I can maintain forever. Fasting will give you quick weight-loss results, and when you return to eating throughout the day, after fasting, that weight will return. You may need to fast at times for religious reasons, and, in this case, I recommend that you eat up until the last minute before your fasting period begins, and then break your fast as soon as you can to avoid long periods of time without food. Just ask yourself what you can do forever as a lifestyle change, and what fuel you need in your body for the best workout.

Do genetics play a factor?

Your genes determine your body type and how you process food. However, there is a chance that you may not get a particular gene from your family member. Your physical appearance is determined in part by what your parents, and even extended family, look like, so even with proper nutrition and exercise, your genetics will still play a part in how you look, your physical ability, and your bone structure.

What foods are good to have when it's "that time of the month"?

We women often deal with three to seven days a month when we can completely lose ourselves in chocolate, salty foods, and tears. It's no joke trying to find balance around this time every single month—your hormones are raging, your belly is bloated, you're starving, and you want to demolish a whole Domino's pizza. Cravings are going to be much higher around this period (no pun intended!), which means you'll need to be even more disciplined. Know what is coming and be prepared. Do your weekly shopping and meal prep beforehand so you have all the healthy options in the fridge ready to go.

The bloat is real! One day you'll have a flat tummy and the next you'll look like you are expecting. This is normal, so don't beat yourself up; just use these tricks to help reduce bloating:

- **Lemon water.** You'll retain less fluid when you flush your system with H2O, so let hydrating lemon water do the job of flushing excess sodium from your body to reduce bloat.
- **Ginger.** This root has anti-inflammatory properties proven to help with "gastric emptying," so if you're bloated because

you haven't made a visit to the loo for a while, try a couple of ginger shots.

- **Lentils.** Hungry for a substantial meal? Lentils are the bomb! They're packed with natural fiber, protein, and complex carbohydrates.
- **Probiotics.** Taking a high-quality daily probiotic supplement can improve gut health and optimize digestive tract function. You can also get the benefits of probiotics from unsweetened yogurt, fermented drinks like kombucha and kefir, or fermented foods such as kimchi and sauerkraut.

What's the best way to get all your veggies in?

Just do it! We are so lucky to have these amazing foods at our fingertips. Vegetables are good for you; you're not five years old anymore and can't cross your arms and say, "I don't like it!" We are big girls and boys now, and we are grateful for nutritious foods that make us smart and powerful. Add them into smoothies; make sure each of your main meals has a healthy serving or two of veggies; keep eating it until you like it; try them all; mix them together; and add some hummus dip! There is no excuse for adults not to get their veggies in if they want to live long and healthy lives. If you are going to keep complaining and absolutely won't get those veggies in, you can add "green" supplements to your meals in the form of powders or tablets.

How much fruit should I eat?

Fruit is like candy from nature! It's candy that has a lot of natural sugar, fiber, vitamins, and minerals. Fruit is a healthy alternative to satisfy that sweet tooth, so it's okay to indulge. That being said, if your body has a difficult time processing sugar, then you should limit your intake. If you do not have any dietary restrictions, three servings of fruit per day are part of a healthy lifestyle. Fruits that are lower in sugar include lemons, limes, grapefruit, berries, cherries, avocado, and honeydew.

What is the most important meal of the day?

Breakfast! I say this because what you eat dictates your mood and energy, so start your day off right with good nutrition and fuel. A healthy breakfast can help boost your metabolism and stabilize your blood sugar levels. Eat within thirty minutes of waking up to get your body going. It is best, though, to skip breakfast if your only choice is something unhealthy, such as doughnuts or fried foods. It's better to begin with nothing rather than simple carbs, sugar, and unhealthy fats. In this case, it's worth waiting until you can get your hands on something good for your body. Traveling with an extra bag of almonds or a protein bar can be a temporary fix—in an emergency situation only!

Are there any foods out there that help boost your metabolism?

Protein-rich foods like chicken, turkey, nuts, eggs, soy, legumes, and fish are great sources. Protein makes you feel full, which can help reduce cravings. Protein will help maintain your body mass and help rebuild muscle.

Citrus fruits are easy to digest and low in sugar. Grapefruit and lemons are rich in vitamin C, which helps your body burn fat faster. Berries help manage glucose levels and decrease body fat. Ginger is often helpful to control your appetite.

How do I pick the right foods at a restaurant?

This could be one of the biggest challenges when trying to get results, especially if you are with people who are not on the same journey as you. Try to order first! Look at the menu, see what is on your nutrition plan, and order quickly so you won't be tempted by what others are ordering.

Restaurant portions are more food than you need, so ask for a takeout container right away, divide your plate in two before you begin eating, and take that extra portion home. Now you have lunch for the next day!

Scan the menu for foods that are grilled or baked. Choose a healthy protein, add your sides of veggies (hold the butter!), ask for the sauce or salad dressing on the side, add some complex carbs, and keep your hands out of the bread basket if you plan to have dessert. It's all about balance—you can't always have your cake and eat it, too, so choose your indulgences wisely. I always tell my clients, "Let's get to where you want to be first with a treat once a week, and once you have achieved that goal, see how you feel." Often the healthy habit is created, and they don't want more than one cheat meal a week!

Can I drink coffee?

Coffee is fine in moderation as long as you are not adding in creamer and sugar, which is where the unwanted calories that lead to weight gain creep in. And don't get me going on all the variations of lattes and cappuccinos you can now get on every street corner! The best solution for energy is food, not caffeine, so be sure to have a healthy breakfast in the morning. I am from England, so obviously I prefer to drink tea! I have switched to thermogenic herbal tea, which gives me energy and includes antioxidants. We've created a culture in which people are monsters before they get their coffee, so if you can't bear to go through life without it, just make sure it's not loaded with extra items. Straight black coffee will do the trick. Coffee is rich in omega 3s, antioxidants, and the vitamins A, K, D, and E; however, it's *not* a substitute for a healthy meal for breakfast. Stick to two cups a day and increase your water intake.

How many calories should I eat per day?

The answer to this question depends on a lot of factors. To simply maintain body weight, women should eat about 2,000 calories per day, while men need about 2,500. Typically, to lose weight women should aim for 1,500 calories per day to lose one pound per week. Everyone is different depending on their personal health and fitness level and the goals they want to achieve. I don't get too caught up with counting my calories. I know that when I am following my meal plan, I am on track with the amount of calories I should be consuming. For me, counting my protein is more important, as that's what gets me through the day, keeps me full, and builds lean muscle. If you're just counting calories, you'll choose a diet soda with zero calories over a tuna steak that is 200 calories because it has less, yet which one is better for you?

What do electrolytes do?

Electrolytes help deliver the water you drink to your muscles more quickly, which helps with your performance while exercising. Electrolytes are essential salts that your body needs to have a chemical reaction with the water in our body. They regulate the flow of water in and out of cells, which is important during physical activity, keeping you focused, hydrated, and able to perform.

What foods are good to improve energy?

The best way to get energy is to have a balanced diet that includes lean protein, complex carbs, good fats, veggies, and water.

A balanced, healthy diet and exercise are what is going to give you energy. There is no magic pill that can wake you up without all the other elements of a great, nutritious diet. The best way to have energy is to have a protein-rich breakfast with healthy carbs and fats, eat regular meals and snacks, stay away from processed foods, get some exercise in, drink water, limit alcohol, and get your necessary vitamins and minerals.

Does my body need sugar?

Yes, your body needs sugar to survive. However, I'm not talking about the sugary food that's just sweet to the taste buds. Your body needs carbohydrates, which are broken down into sugar in your body. This sugar is essential for your body to create energy to survive. It is interesting to me that people question the amount of sugar in shakes and then go eat a banana, which has more sugar. Sugar also helps your body deliver protein to your muscles so it can grow and repair. Choose healthy carbs from whole grains, fruits, and veggies, and you'll take in all the sugar you need.

Should I count macros?

The good news is that I do not measure my food on a scale, and I have still been able to maintain a healthy physique. You can definitely get results by doing this method, and if it works for you, go for it. Personally, I find that it's time consuming and doesn't always mean you're getting all the nutrients for an optimal and healthy diet. The recipes in this book have been formulated to a target macro of approximately 40 percent carbs, 30 percent protein, and 30 percent fat. This is a basic guideline to follow when creating your meals and planning.

Can I have cheat days?

This is up to you! If you want the best shot at achieving your goals, I wouldn't be going out and eating cake. Rather than a whole cheat day (because that's a little excessive), have a cheat meal once in a while. Build your cheat meal into your weekly routine, enjoy it, and get back on plan.

Tasks

- Identify the first item that you are going to cut out for the next thirty days that is not helping you with your results.
- If you drink alcohol, track your intake for the next fourteen days and see if this is helping you get the results you are working for.
- Note what triggers your stress eating and what foods you gravitate toward. When you have these feelings, use the tools you have learned from this chapter to navigate yourself to a healthier choice and move your body.

7

Building a Training Schedule

I work out for a break, for my health, and to push myself physically. I even work out to get away from my phone! (Otherwise I swear by age forty I will have a claw hand and be unable to text!)

I also work out just because it makes me feel good. It's super fun when you have found what you like. For me, filming the videos for my audience is the best thing ever. I chat with them through it and push myself because I want to lead by example.

Everyone's schedule is totally different, so what might work for one person will be a terrible idea for someone else. This is why I created my fitness and nutrition app that can be used at home with minimal equipment, doesn't require a bunch of ingredients, and is suitable for all levels.

The ultimate training schedule is, of course, my 30-Day Level Up Challenge (Chapter 9). If you want to build a long-term schedule, I know that you are going to have a couple of questions, so to make it easy and set you up for future success, here are the answers.

Fitness Q&A

What is the best time to work out?

Different studies show benefits at all hours of the day. Instead of worrying about what time to do it, just do it! If you only have time in the morning, great; if you only have time in the evening, also great! I do notice when I train later on in the day that I have more energy and power, because I have more fuel in my body from food that increases my performance. In the morning I can be slower and I don't have the energy reserves to hit a personal best.

Can I double up on my workouts?

If you miss a day, it's okay. Keep missing lots of days in a row and then Houston, we have a problem! The longer you're away from it, the more trouble you will face getting into the swing of things and back on track. You know how your body feels, so if you skipped a workout the day before and today you feel like you can add in some extra reps, then go for it. (Not at the risk of injury or fatigue, though!)

How often should I have a rest day?

Your body has to rest to get results, so whatever you do, rest days are a must. Decide what day works best for you and make that your rest day. On your rest day (or two), I suggest stretching and a very light walk to keep your body mobile.

Can I work out on my period? When is the best time in my menstrual cycle to work out?

Ahh, it's that time of the month! You just cussed out your boyfriend, cried in your car for no reason, and *now* you have to work out?! Getting motivated on your period is hard work . . . ugh, hormones! The big question is: Can you work out on your period?

Well, yes! Everyone has a unique period and we all experience hormonal changes differently. Learn the ways to stick to your healthy lifestyle during every phase of your menstrual cycle. Your brain might be telling your body "NO"—you can break free from this! Let's break it down week by week, girls. Here's how to manage your monthly cycle to maximize your results.

Days 1–5.

The first day of your menstrual cycle is the first day of your period. Welcome to the food-craving phase—you probably want to pick up that pint of ice cream here! That's normal. Your estrogen is slowly rising; the initial dip in hormones means that your body will let you shed fat faster compared to the rest of the month! Surprisingly, this stage of the menstrual cycle is ideal to *push* yourself.

During this time, you'll probably feel like crap! Try low-impact exercises like yoga, light cardio, and swimming. Movement can help reduce cramping and headaches, so let's release those endorphins to boost our mood. Some women might build a tolerance for pain during the first half of their period, so see if working out makes you feel better!

Days 6–13.

Hello, testosterone! Testosterone is your friend when building muscle. At this time of the month you'll feel motivated and energized. You'll have higher levels of hormones that will make you want to sprint or take on more weight-training exercises.

This is a great time to get in whatever challenges you the most! Whether it's weight training, cardio, or whatever, this time is when you'll have that drive to complete those exercises. Give it a go!

Days 14–21.

Now you've entered the ovulation phase. At this time of the month you might feel sluggish: Your estrogen is starting to dip and progesterone is starting to rise. This is a cocktail to promote fat-burning abilities.

It's time to get your heart rate up! Exercises such as running and Pilates are light enough to keep your body engaged and burning calories. If you can't break through your lethargic stage, try going on a nature walk or a bike ride.

Days 21–28.

Ahh, the calm before the storm. Or maybe the pre-storm? You'll be feeling "blah" this week! Estrogen and testosterone take a dive and you'll start to bloat. Yes, everyone bloats! Try not to get discouraged (and see pages 102–103 for tips to beat the bloat!).

This week is a good time for steady cardio, body workouts, and yoga. You'll stay active and combat some classic symptoms of PMS.

Girls, you know your body, and guys, this might be the opportunity for you to get out of the house and go to the gym. Or even better, try one of my ab workouts together and see what these girls are made of!

When should I increase my weights?

If you have been using the same weights for the past thirty to sixty days, it's time to increase those "lbs," and no, you're not going to bulk up! The last few reps of your exercise should be challenging, so if you are flying through those last two to three reps, it's time to up those bad boys.

Should I work out if I am sore?

If your legs are sore, work your arms instead. You don't need to work out an area of your body that is in recovery; there are plenty of other parts from which to choose.

What if I have an injury?

Working out hard on an injury is like putting fuel in the fire—you are only going to make it worse. Add in a lot of stretching and light movement to keep your body agile and loose. If you are concerned, go see a health practitioner who can assess you in person.

What if I have a previous commitment, like a vacation?

This is called life! If you have the BURN workout app you can take it everywhere, even without Wi-Fi! If you don't, write out some of your favorite workouts from a class or YouTube video and take them with you. Remember, there are no excuses, and you have the perfect chance to implement that rule here!

Commit to sticking to your workout on vacation. Pack some resistance bands, take a hike, look for a fitness class at your resort or the community where you're staying, or hit the water to swim and snorkel. Make sure to send me a postcard or an Instagram photo of you working out on vacation so I can give you a high five for making it happen for yourself!

Should I stick to the same workout?

Ideally, no. Mix it up, keep it interesting, shock your body to wake up different muscles, try something new, and get out of your comfort zone. On the other hand, if you dislike exercising and find something you love, then keep doing it. Want to know what workout to do? The one you *will do*!

What will happen if I skip a workout?

If you skip one workout, don't beat yourself up. If you work out twice a week and eat the proper nutrition, you will see results; it'll just take you longer than if you're eating the same way and working out four or five times a week.

If you do skip a workout, be conscious of what you're eating, and don't sneak in that doughnut. Even getting ten minutes of exercise a day is better than doing nothing at all, as you are still moving your body. Use it or lose it!

4 Tips to Prepare for a Workout

You're about set for a workout, and you might not be feeling ready, confident, or in the mood. Yet you have results to gain so you're going to get that workout in! Use these tips to get you fired up to take action.

1. **Freshen your breath.**
   We are breathing all the time when we are exercising. You don't want the taste of an old taco or milkshake halfway through your burpee! Plus, that minty fresh feel wakes us up.

2. **Don the right gear.**
   What are you going to wear? You want to feel good in your outfit, so choose clothes that make you feel motivated and are appropriate for the style of workout you are doing. You don't want your boobs to make an appearance because you're doing skater hops in a loose-fitting bra!

3. **Set up your time.**
   If you're going to the gym for a class, get there with enough time to get the equipment you need for your routine. If you're doing a workout from home, let people know that this is your sacred "feel the burn time" and they are not to interrupt.

4. **Hydrate.**
   I like to put electrolytes in my water because it gets to my muscles faster for a more powerful workout. Always have a water bottle nearby when you are working out, and keep it filled up. Twenty minutes before I start to exercise, I take a pre-workout electrolyte supplement. I just put the powder straight in my mouth and chug it with some water. It's pretty gnarly, so be prepared if you try it!

5 Moves to Boost Your Energy

If there are days when you really feel like you can't get motivated, remember that there are no excuses, so commit to moving your body for at least ten minutes a day. Do these energy-boosting moves when you're feeling down and need a pick-me-up to get your day started or when you need a little help getting over the afternoon slump. You might have to walk outside your office or do it under your desk. Your coworkers might look at you like you're weird, yet they will thank you later after you wake up and become more productive.

Do each one for thirty seconds and repeat through twice. If you are feeling it, just keep on going.

1. **Plank in-and-out jumps:** Start in a plank position, either a high plank or on your forearms, with feet together. Jump your feet out about two feet apart, then jump back in.

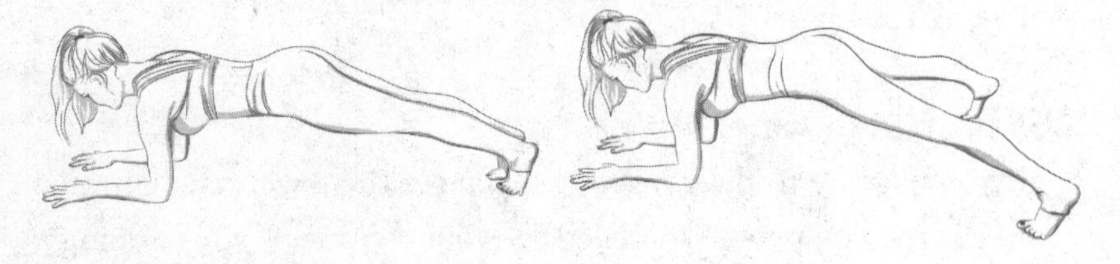

2. **Split lunges:** Start in a split stance, right foot forward, left foot back. Bend your legs so your back knee nearly touches the floor, then extend through both legs and jump, switching legs in the air. Land softly with your knees bent, left foot forward, right foot back. Jump again to switch to the other side.

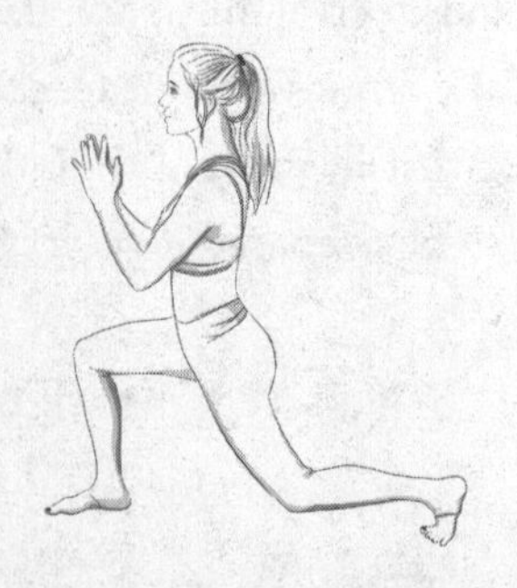

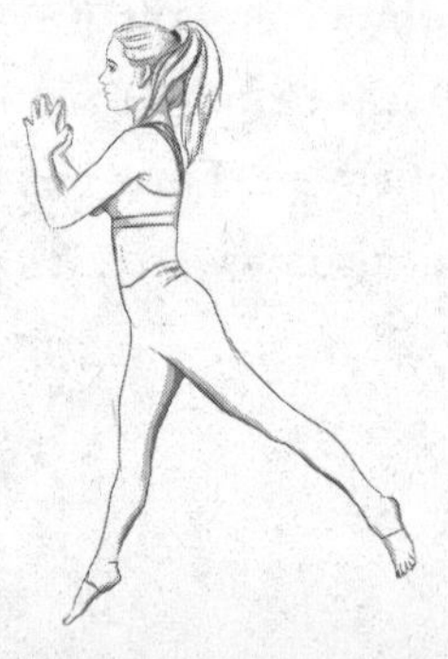

3. **Charlie's angels:** Lunge forward, bring your arms in front, and twist to your front leg. Alternate from your left to your right.

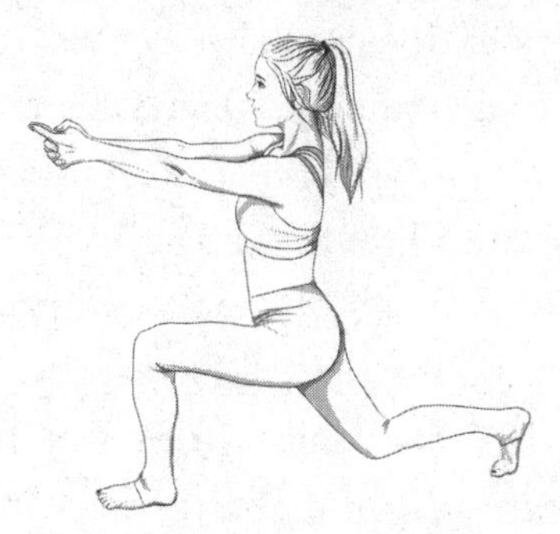

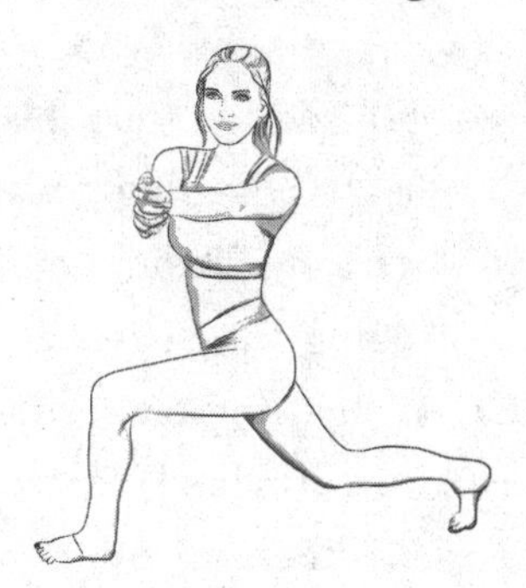

4. **V-sit or boat pose:** Lie down on your back with your arms over your head. Use your arms for momentum to sit up. Hold with your legs bent out in front and arms straight in front of you. Slowly go back down to the ground.

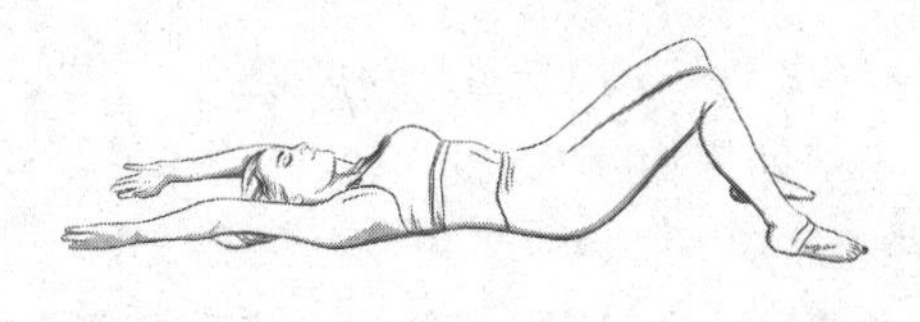

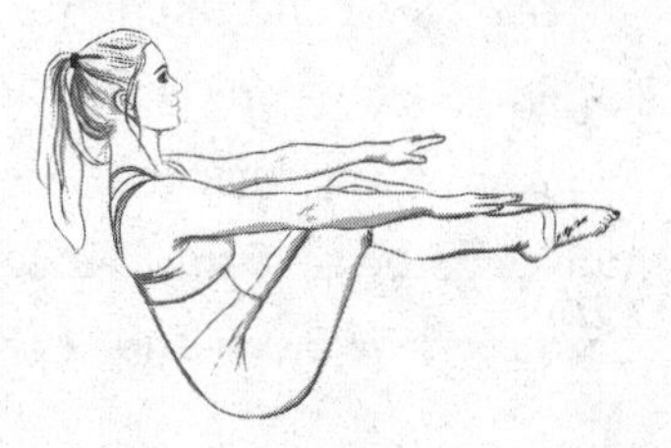

5. **High knees:** Bring your knees up to your chest one at a time as high as you can. To make it more challenging, speed it up and get your heart rate going to release those endorphins.

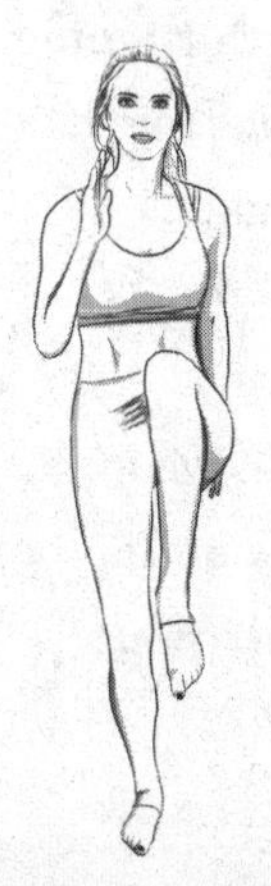

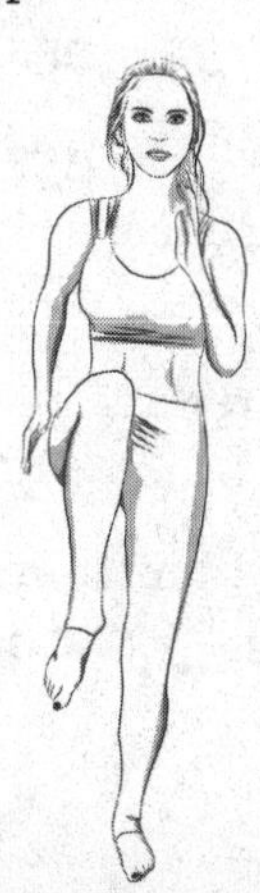

What Burns More Calories?

We all want to know exactly how many calories we burn every single minute of the day. At least this was my train of thought when I obsessed over exercise and eating. I wanted to know exactly what I had burned off on the treadmill and therefore how much I could eat that day. After years of doing this, I realized this full-time job of counting calories wasn't even getting me results. I used to think that all I needed to do was run, run, run it all off, yet I really didn't like running too much. The good news is there are other ways you can burn off the extra cookie that don't involve a treadmill!

Cardio.
Cardio is great for getting your heart rate up and strengthening your cardiovascular system. Since it makes your heart beat faster, more oxygen and nutrients are carried to your cells. Try biking, jogging, swimming, HIIT (high-intensity interval training) workouts, and my cardio videos. If you are looking to lose weight, you're going to want to incorporate cardio into your workout, as cardio burns more calories during exercise than strength training.

Strength training.
Strength training involves various moves in which you are lifting weights. When you lift light weights, you are activating different muscle fibers than you do when you lift heavy weights, so it's good to switch it up. The great thing about strength training is that once you're done, you will continue to burn calories for the rest of the day, which means it's also great for losing weight!

For optimal results, overall fitness, and good health—do both!

How do you know what you are capable of? Well, you don't know until you try! I hit a personal best of hip thrusts of 355 pounds, which is a lot more than my body weight of around 107 pounds. While I had no idea what I could do until I started doing it, my mind didn't limit me from seeing what was possible. All I did was show up each week, fuel my body with good food, thrust what my trainer told me to, and not quit. As time went on and I was consistent, it became easier and easier to lift the next level of weights. When you try to do ten times more than what you think you can do, everything less becomes so much easier. After lifting 355 pounds, I could rep 95 pounds all day long! My body had learned what it was like at that level, adapted, and grown to where it needed to be to support the weight. Just like in your mindset, you must "ten-times" your thinking so that the big things don't seem so huge, and you are now able to deal with situations that at one time might have been impossible to solve. See how far you can go, and then go some more!

Body Goals

Let's talk about #Bodygoals! Yes, I have them, and I am always looking to improve. There are days when I am not as motivated to work out, then I take a quick glance at how my results are doing and I think to myself either that I am on a roll here and I need to keep going, or okay, it's time to get back on it and go to the gym. Either way there is motivation right there to go be active and get a sweat on. I realized that looking at myself in the mirror to compare myself or point out my flaws doesn't do anything apart from make me feel like shit. So, I stopped doing that and instead spent that time doing a workout that I love. We are always on this journey, and trust me, every day I feel like I can do more, just thinking about that perfectly round perky butt that I want. And at the same time, I am content with where I am—coming from a place of gratitude—while pursuing where I want to go.

Only you can decide the results you want. Maybe you are looking for a happy medium, to be in okay shape, be healthy, and still enjoy the occasional cocktail and treat. It goes back to what is important to you. This is your choice and ultimately you have control of your success.

Cool Down and Recovery

It's important to cool down and recover both after your workout and in life itself! I can work all day and all night—I have no "off button." When I started to take better care of myself and forced myself to switch off, I became a better and nicer person to be around. Riled up, stressed out, and pissed off, then having to interact with other human beings? Recipe for disaster! Take yourself away to unwind and come back to neutral. This needs to be done before you get to your boiling point. Have an escape plan in place so you remain calm when situations get tough.

My "me time" can be as simple as taking the dogs for a walk, getting out in the fresh air, and putting my phone in my pocket. I heard that weekly massages were a must for giving your body love, and I wasn't going to argue with that. Now I will go for the occasional massage; I can't have my phone in there, so I am forced to disconnect. Plus it feels darn good, too!

One of my favorite ten-minute breaks is to simply sit with some hot tea, and a little chocolate, and enjoy the moment of not doing anything. This is what starts that fire again in my stomach and how I am able to sustain the speed at which I work and get things done. It's essential to book these little breaks into your week—they are just as important as the work itself because this is work on you. The times when you are relaxing and unwinding is when you have the most clarity, so give your brain time to ease down on a daily basis. It's not only going to help you—it will help everyone around you. However, the relaxation time can't be more time than the work—let's make that clear!

Here are my favorite exercises to unwind and give my body self-care. Spend fifteen to twenty minutes doing these stretches every day if you can. Aim for at least two to three stretch sessions a week to feel the benefits of loosening up your body. Hold each pose for thirty to forty seconds. When a pose feels good, feel free to stay there; this is not to be rushed, so look after your body.

Exercises for Stretching and Relaxing

Pigeon **Downward-facing dog**

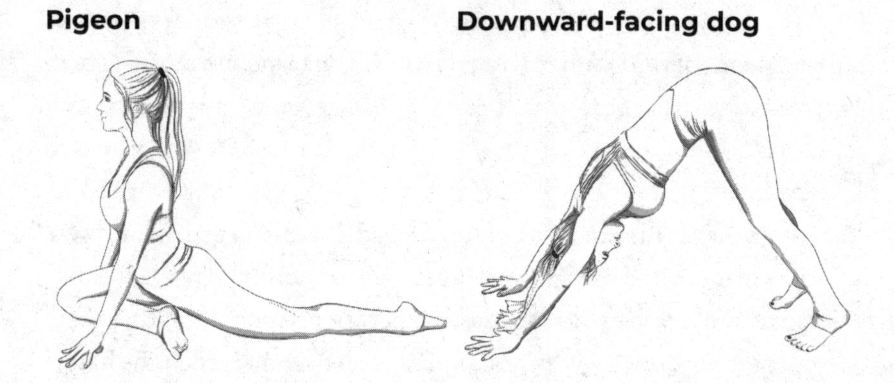

Cobra **Seated forward fold**

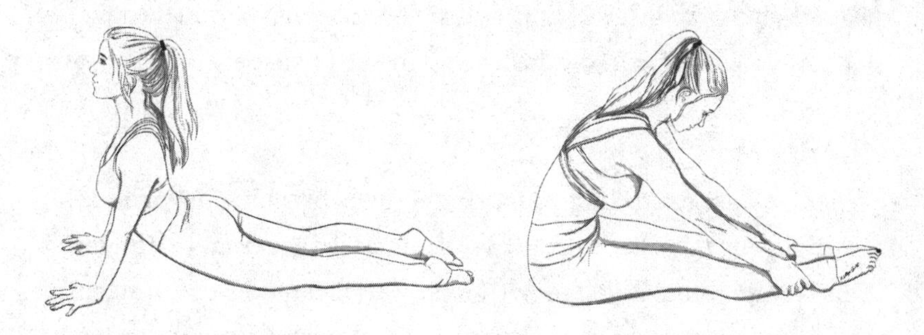

Supine twist

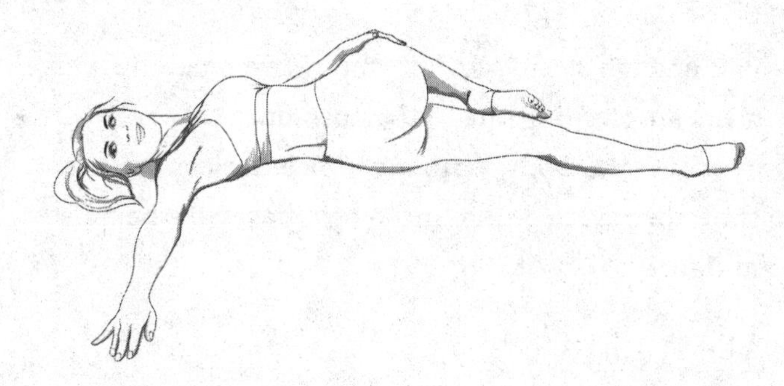

Recovery

Recovery is an essential part of getting results both physically and in life. Whether you are sore from exercise, had a long day, or are just feeling the weight of the world on your shoulders, incorporate these ways to get you back to peak performance and to being a happy, positive person.

Ice bath.

Dr. Trisha Smith explains how an ice bath has many benefits for you both mentally, to control your breath and mind, and physically, to repair and recover your muscles. It's best to just go for it rather than taking your time to get in. As soon as you're submerged in the bath, the goal is to calm your breathing and get into a meditative state. When we work out, we tear down the muscles in our body. Cold water helps to reduce swelling and speed recovery, so you'll come back to your next workout faster and in better shape.

Nutrition.

When you are exercising you are effectively breaking down and tearing your muscles so that they grow back bigger and stronger. This is impossible if you're not feeding your muscles the nutrients and ingredients they need to respire. Replenish your muscles with balanced nutrition to build muscle and speed up recovery time.

Sleep.

You have to have enough sleep. Most of your tissue repair happens at night when you are sleeping due to the hormones that are pumping throughout your body. Without sufficient sleep, you're not going to show up to your workout the next day with the most power and endurance.

Rest.

Take a day or two off from your workouts a week to let your body heal. Working out and getting results is a process, and resting is one of the steps you must take to see results. If you keep tearing your muscles apart, you're not going to allow them time to come together and repair. The American College of Sports Medicine recommends that you train each major muscle group two or three days per week and allow forty-eight hours of recovery between the different areas that you work out. This is exactly why I created my training program, so that you have a schedule of exactly what workouts to do, allowing you to follow along in the comfort of your own home.

Massage.

Having many beneficial properties, touch is great for your body. A 2008 study by researchers at The Ohio State University discovered that Swedish massage helps the muscles recover faster with less evidence of swelling and inflammation. Bestselling author Robin Sharma told me that he books in weekly massages as part of his routine so that he can be the most productive in his work. Just taking that time for ourselves can often give us more creativity and calmness, making us much nicer to be around. Look after you first so you can be the best role model for others.

Tasks

- Write down a list of at least three types of exercise or workouts that you love. Doing this will jumpstart that positive feeling when you think of exercise!
- What new style of workout are you going to try this week? Look in your local area for classes that you have not tried before and book one. Go on YouTube, find a new workout style, and give it a go. You never

know what you might like unless you try it. You don't know what you don't know!

- Track your sleep for the next week. Are you getting in at least seven hours a night? This might be an opportunity to reflect and see how you can get to bed earlier to give your body enough time to rest and recover.

PART III

THE 30-DAY LEVEL UP CHALLENGE

8

Creating Your New Routine

Routines keep you organized, and when you're organized, you will stay on track. Creating a structure for your day is one of the most crucial parts of your success, and in this chapter we are going to set you up with everything you need to complete the challenge and level up your life!

Ready for Success

In the 30-Day Level Up Challenge, you'll be making changes to every part of your life—your mindset, your meals, your fitness routine, and so much more. Are you ready? Hopefully, you've begun by making small changes as you worked your way through the book, and if not, there's no time like right now! Let's take those first steps to prepare for the challenge.

Is your kitchen filled with junk food, like sugary snacks and chips? Get rid of them now so you won't have to deal with temptation later. Clean out the refrigerator to make room for the healthy meals you'll be prepping, and stock up on everything you need so that when the time comes to begin the plan, all you have to do is shop for perishable foods, prep your meals, and get going! If you share a refrigerator with roommates or family, make sure you have a section set aside just for you, so that you can store your prepped meals and snacks without having to rummage through food that isn't on the plan.

Pantry Shopping and Supplies

Before you begin, make sure you have all of the pantry staples and supplies you will need to cook and store your food, do your workouts, and complete your daily tasks. Shop for these items before you begin the challenge—having all of your shelf-stable items and frequently used produce on hand when you begin will make your weekly shopping trips easier. Get ready to shop!

Staple Items

Almond butter (1 jar)
Almonds, sliced (1 ounce plus more for snacks if desired)
Artichoke hearts, water-packed (two 14-ounce cans)
Baking powder
Bread, 100% whole wheat (1 loaf, freeze half)
Canned beans (15-ounce cans): black beans (6 cans), chickpeas (2 cans), navy beans (1 can), pinto beans (2 cans)
Cashews, raw (one 8-ounce container)
Coconut, dried unsweetened (1 bag)
Coconut milk, light (one 14-ounce can)
Coconut water (two 8-ounce containers)
Cranberries, dried (1 package)

Medjool dates, pitted (one 8-ounce container)
Dijon mustard
Grains: quinoa (1 container), brown rice (1 container), whole wheat pastry flour (1 small bag)
Granola, lightly sweetened (1 bag)
Honey, raw (1 jar)
Hot sauce, your favorite (1 bottle)
Kalamata olives, pitted (1 jar)
Oils: coconut oil, extra-virgin olive oil, toasted sesame oil
Pasta: whole wheat penne (1 package)
Produce: carrots, garlic, lemons, yellow onions
Protein powder (your favorite brand, vanilla flavor)
Reduced-sodium soy sauce (1 bottle)
Rolled oats (1 container)
Salad dressing: Asian ginger vinaigrette
Seeds: chia seeds, hemp seeds
Spices, dried: chili powder, cumin, Italian seasoning, oregano, red pepper flakes, thyme
Thai green curry paste (1 jar)
Tomatoes, canned: diced (one 14.5-ounce can), whole peeled plum (four 14.5-ounce cans)
Tuna, canned white (two 5-ounce cans)
Vinegars: apple cider vinegar, balsamic vinegar

Supplies

Food storage containers.
Make sure you have plenty of glass or BPA-free plastic storage containers in a variety of sizes. You'll need meal-size containers for storing prepped meals; pint- or quart-size containers for storing prepped items such as brown rice, quinoa, and hard-boiled eggs; and small containers for sauces and condiments. Mason jars are great for fridge storage, and for the freezer, you'll want plastic or a temperature-safe glass like Pyrex. Pick up some plastic wrap

and baggies in a variety of sizes, or buy eco-friendly beeswax wrap to cover bowls and wrap sandwiches.

Kitchen equipment.

Most of the recipes in this book can be prepared with the equipment you already have in your kitchen. You'll need saucepans and sauté pans/skillets with lids in a variety of sizes; a large nonstick pan; a mesh strainer; large, rimmed baking sheets; spoons and spatulas; and a food processor or blender. A slow cooker is nice to have though not essential—anything you can cook in a slow cooker can also be cooked on the stovetop. Parchment paper helps to keep food from sticking when you're roasting those veggies, and it makes cleanup a snap, too.

Essential workout equipment.

You'll need a yoga mat, a towel, and a water bottle. A set of resistance bands and weights are optional, and don't forget to bring a massive smile! And never underestimate the power of a quality sports bra!

Writing supplies.

Get yourself a notebook for journaling, Post-it notes, and some colorful pens—choose colors and textures that make you happy! You'll also need poster paper, scissors, craft glue, and any "extras" that appeal to you for making inspirational signs, affirmations, vision boards, and more.

Morning Affirmations

Even if you feel silly, it's important to start your day with positive reinforcement. Get in front of your mirror, look dead on at yourself, change your physiological state by standing up tall, and say with conviction your daily affirmations. Stick to one each day and repeat until you believe what you are saying inside. It might take ten minutes the first time to even have the guts to say anything out loud, and it's probably going to feel incredibly uncomfortable. Remember, we grow in times of being uncomfortable, so let yourself go and scream it out; it will become second nature to you in time.

Task

- Write out your daily affirmations. Make a list of as many affirmations as you can think of and pick a different one each day to say to yourself in the mirror in the morning. Say each one a good four or five times to make sure you are listening and taking it to heart.

I've included a schedule of sample affirmations below; you can of course create your own and make them whatever you need them to be!

Monday: My ability to conquer challenges is limitless; my potential to succeed is infinite.

Tuesday: I will not compare myself to others.

Wednesday: Today, I abandon my old habits and take up new, more positive ones.

Thursday: I am in charge of how I feel today, and I am choosing happiness.

Friday: Every experience is contributing to my growth.

Saturday: All that I need comes to me at the right time and place in this life.

Sunday: I can. I will.

Your Morning Routine

Create your own morning routine that fits into what you want to achieve from the advice below. Take time to hydrate, eat a healthy meal, stretch, reflect, and set the tone for the day ahead. Write it out in timed blocks to keep you on track. Starting with a set time frame really helps when you feel like you are crunched for time. And if you really want to have it all, go to bed earlier! You will be much more productive in the morning.

Here are some key elements that you want to add into your morning routine to set you up for a successful day:

Use an alarm clock.

Yep, it all starts with how you wake up. Those terrible ones on our phones startle us, waking us up in a panic. Get an alarm clock that slowly wakes you up with birds chirping and brings light into the room. Trust me, this is magic. And don't snooze! Institute the "five-second rule": when your alarm goes off, count down from five and then immediately get up. Hitting snooze and going back to sleep is only going to throw off your schedule, make you more tired, mess up your sleep patterns, and have you off center before the day even begins.

Set the mood.

Whether you have kids or not, you'll want to set aside at least twenty minutes that are just for you every morning. My dogs are so lazy that they sometimes don't get up until 10 AM, so I can't at this moment relate to those of you who have mini people waking you up. Getting up before them to have your own space to breathe is critical. Taking this time for yourself sets you up for success and helps you manage your stress levels and reactions throughout the day.

Light a candle, burn some incense, or diffuse some essential oils—a pleasant-smelling environment will help you to feel relaxed. Play some music or peaceful sounds—I use a calming app to play ocean sounds. Add some good natural light—nothing too bright and alarming, just enough to begin waking you up. Doesn't this sound really nice? Yes! And your behavior through the day is going to be a lot calmer and more productive in a positive way when you are aligned from the moment you wake up.

Fuel yourself.

You need brain power and physical energy, which means eating a nutrient-rich breakfast. Coffee is a no-go straightaway in the morning. When you wake up, you're slightly dehydrated, and coffee will only make things worse. Start with a big glass of water with lemon or aloe to get your body in working order. Then eat your breakfast, which is the most important meal of the day when you do it right.

Move your body for five to ten minutes.

This is not your workout for the day; it's simply to get your joints loose, help wake you up, and stop you from going back to sleep. Stretch, do some yoga, or have a dance party—do whatever you feel you need that day to get going. Just move around!

Read for personal development.

You've set the mood for the day, hydrated yourself, moved around, and eaten a solid breakfast to create energy, and now it's time to fill up that mind with some positive stuff. You are going to get all kinds of shit thrown at you today. Do you want it to bounce off you or consume your energy?

Getting ten to fifteen minutes of reading into your day first thing in the morning, before your "world buzzer" goes off, is essential to owning your day. Personal development books are game changers. I like to read rather than listen to audiobooks, because it's easy to get distracted and think you can multitask, which is the biggest misconception about productivity. Stick to ten to fifteen minutes—any more than that can be too much information, and you'll want to apply what you've learned before you move on to the next chapter. Read a little and put it into practice, and if you feel you need to, read the same content for a couple of days until it really sinks into your brain.

Yep, this can seem like a lot to do first thing in the morning. Really, how are you going to succeed in life if you can't even get your shit together in the morning? This might take you an hour the first time to get it all in order; however, once you put this into daily practice, you can get it down to thirty minutes.

If you are already saying, "I can't do this, Rebecca," I have an answer: That's BS. You have to make it happen. If you can't take thirty minutes for yourself to be a good human for the rest of the day, you might need to re-think your priorities. Remember, everything is a choice, and you can choose to take responsibility and make this happen, with no excuses. Find your "why," set your alarm to get up thirty minutes earlier, and do it!

Your Nighttime Routine

Just as you start your day with a routine, you'll also want to create an evening ritual that will end your day on a positive note so you can have a great night's sleep. It is important to start winding down one or two hours before you are about to hit the pillow to fall asleep. If I don't do this, I'll lie in bed thinking about things, with my brain going around like a hamster wheel. Does this sound familiar to you? Then it's time to end your day with a new routine.

Turn off electronics a few hours before you go to bed. Put your phone down (for real) and turn off the television. These forms of entertainment stimulate your brain and create a stress response, and it takes a while to calm down. Dim the lights, read a little, write in your journal, or do a little meal prep and choose an outfit for the next day—set yourself up for a good night's sleep and a stress-free morning.

Enjoy a snack, relaxing tea, and/or supplements.

I like to have my last protein snack around this time along with a natural tea supplement, which helps to settle me down for a good night's sleep.

Wash away the day.

End your day with a warm shower, then do your skin care routine, such as makeup removal followed by a wash, toner, and night cream. Taking good care of your skin is an essential part of good self-care. Feeling clean and cozy as I get into bed helps me to fall asleep quickly.

Breathe and relax.

Once you get into bed, get comfortable and breathe deeply—you've earned a rest! When I am really struggling to sleep, I will use a meditation or a story from an app like Calm. When you listen to the words of someone else, your thoughts are not flying through your head at a million miles an hour.

Express gratitude.

Just before I fall asleep, I take a moment to write in my gratitude journal. Jot down three great things that happened that day, and what you could have done to make it a better day. This is a sealing off of the day, leaving you feeling thankful for the life you have and ready to face whatever comes next.

Tasks

- Sit down with your diary and schedule your morning and evening routines in detail.
- Get ready to start the 30-Day Level Up Challenge. Shop for your pantry items, get your workout gear together, and set yourself up for success!

9

The 30-Day Level Up Challenge

You've made it this far, and I couldn't be prouder of you! The fact that you picked up this book and chose to read it means you've already taken a step in the right direction. The next challenge you will face is implementing everything you've learned into your daily life and staying consistent with your plan. It's not going to come easy, and when you make a conscious decision every day to focus on breaking old habits then you *will* maximize the results you see on day 30.

Now it's time for some fun: putting it all into practice! You'll be tested during this part, and you're going to use all the tools from the book to make sure you pass each test. Commit to doing the 30-Day Level Up Challenge with me and get excited to use your new mindset to conquer and crush your goals!

Each day you will get a workout to complete, a daily meal plan with breakfast, lunch, and dinner recipes that can all be found in Chapter

11, and snacks (page 140) to keep you from being hungry and help you meet your daily protein goal.

The recipes are mixed up throughout the thirty days to keep it interesting and exciting, and most of them make more than one portion, so you won't have to cook new and different meals every day. Do a big meal prep at the beginning of each week and a smaller prep session mid-week, and you'll be able to grab most of your meals out of the fridge and simply heat them up.

You will find a motivational quote to live by every day. Say it out loud and remind yourself of it while you practice implementing it.

Each day you'll complete tasks that are designed to challenge you and stretch your way of thinking. You'll clean out the things you don't need any more and bring a new, lighter energy into your life!

It's time to use that grit and level up your achievements! Are you ready?! Even if you think you aren't, now is the perfect time. Let's get started with waking up your entire body and feeling alive. Get ready to fuel your body with lots of nutritious food and live a balanced life. You've got this!

Workouts Online

You can find the 30-Day Challenge online with the workout videos at www.rebecca-louise.com/my30daychallenge. Click on "access My 30 Day It Takes Grit Challenge" and enter the code ICANDOTHIS.

DAYS 1–7

Shopping List

Dairy and Protein

Almond milk, ½ gallon

Chicken breast, boneless and skinless (two ½-pound breasts)

Eggs, large (1 dozen)

Feta cheese (1 container)

Fish and seafood: halibut (10 ounces); tuna (two 4-ounce steaks); shrimp, frozen, peeled, and deveined, medium (one 2-pound bag)

Greek yogurt, unsweetened, nonfat (one 35-ounce container)

Parmesan cheese, shredded or grated (1 container)

Provolone cheese, deli-sliced (⅛ pound)

Turkey, ground, 99% lean (12 ounces)

Produce

Apples (2)

Arugula (1 small package or bunch)

Avocado (1)

Baby spinach (one 5-ounce package)

Banana (1)

Bell peppers, red (2)

Berries, your choice, for breakfast side (1 cup)

Blueberries (one 10-ounce container)

Broccoli slaw (1 bag)

Button mushrooms (one 5-ounce container)

Grape tomatoes (one 10-ounce package)

Green beans (6 ounces)

Herbs, fresh: basil (1 large bunch), cilantro (1 bunch), rosemary (1 small package), thyme (1 small package)

Lemon (1)

Limes (2)

Mango (1)

Onion, red (2 medium)

Oranges (2)

Peas, frozen (1 small bag)

Peaches (2 small)

Sweet potato (1)

Zucchini (3)

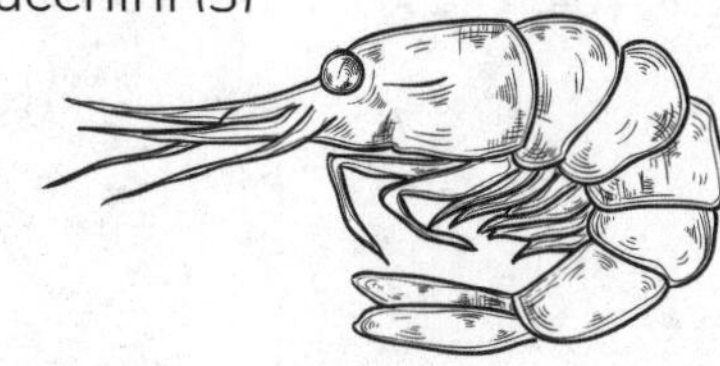

Other

Bread: Whole wheat lavash wraps (use 2, freeze remainder), small whole wheat tortillas (use 4, freeze remainder)

Reduced-sodium vegetable broth (one 32-ounce box)

Grape jelly, all-fruit (one 8-ounce jar)

Nori furikake (1 package; see Kitchen Tip on page 274)

Soba noodles (1 bundle)

Meal Prep Plan

Meal prep is broken down into two days to make it easy for you to always have a mix of fresh and frozen meals ready. If you prefer to do it all on one day, you can put most of these meals in the freezer and then just make your smoothies, fresh fish, and salads as needed.

Day 1: Before you begin, cook 2 hard-boiled eggs (plus more for snacks if you like), 1½ cups brown rice, and 1 cup quinoa—see page 286 for detailed instructions.

Prepare Blueberry Greek Yogurt Pancakes (2 portions in fridge/1 in freezer), Mango Shrimp Tacos (all in fridge), Veggie Lover's Chili (2 portions in fridge/3 in freezer), Blueberry Balsamic Turkey Meatballs (1 portion in fridge/3 in freezer), and Sweet Potato Toast with Avocado and Egg (all in fridge).

Day 5: Prepare Parmesan Veggie Frittata (1 portion in fridge/1 in freezer), Lemon-Herb Chicken Pasta (refrigerate second portion), and grill your chicken for the Grilled Chicken and Peach Salad.

Fresh prep: Unless you have serious time constraints, plan to prepare these meals fresh when you're ready to eat them: Teriyaki Tuna with Roasted Green Beans and Soba (refrigerate the second portion), Reboot Spinach and Almond Butter Smoothie, Pesto Tuna Wraps (can be made the night before), and Halibut and Veggie Skewers (refrigerate the second portion).

Plan your snacks: Choose what appeals to you from the list on pages 140–141, planning for three per day.

Snacks

Plan to eat three snacks each day in addition to your meals. If you do a post-workout shake, make that one of your snacks. (See pages 19–20 for more about post-workout shakes.) Aim for 10 to 15 grams of protein per snack plus healthy carbs and a little fat, and don't forget to keep that water bottle handy and keep sipping!

Healthy Snack Ideas

- Turkey roll-ups: 1 ounce deli turkey, 1 slice provolone cheese, Dijon mustard, apple slices, baby spinach
- 1 hard-boiled egg and ½ cup fresh berries
- Greek yogurt parfait: In a small jar, layer ½ cup unsweetened nonfat Greek yogurt, ½ cup fresh fruit, and 2 tablespoons granola
- Sliced apple and 2 tablespoons almond butter
- ½ cup hummus with raw veggies
- ½ cup cottage cheese with celery
- ½ cup edamame
- Leftovers (half portion)
- 1 No-Bake Lime Coconut Protein Bite (page 249)
- 1 sweet potato toast (page 241) with hummus, avocado mash (page 241), or almond butter
- 1 Blueberry Greek Yogurt Pancake (page 237) with 1 tablespoon almond butter
- 2 ounces tuna, 1 teaspoon each olive oil and lemon juice, and handful of whole grain crackers

- 1 slice whole wheat toast, 1 tablespoon almond butter, and half of a sliced banana
- ½ can tuna
- 100-calorie bag of roasted almonds
- Tomato, basil, and fresh mozzarella
- Protein bites:

  In a medium bowl, mix 6 chopped, pitted Medjool dates, 2 scoops of your favorite protein powder, 2 tablespoons chia seeds, and 4 teaspoons of natural peanut butter.

  Mix well, scoop into golf ball–size portions, and roll in unsweetened dried coconut. Store in the fridge for up to 1 week.
- Roasted chickpeas:

  Preheat your oven to 350°F. Drain and rinse 2 cans of chickpeas, then wrap them gently in a clean kitchen towel to dry them as much as possible.

  Toss the chickpeas on a parchment-lined baking sheet with 1 tablespoon extra-virgin olive oil and your choice of seasonings (a little salt and pepper plus 1 teaspoon chili powder *or* 1 teaspoon each dried Italian seasoning and garlic powder *or* 1 teaspoon each cumin and turmeric).

  Bake until crispy, about 30 minutes, shaking the pan once or twice. Cool completely and store in an airtight container at room temperature.

Day 1

Let's get going and start as we mean to go on! The only person in the way of not completing this 30-Day Level Up Challenge is you. You have the choice!

Failing to prepare is preparing to fail.

Workout: Full Body BURN

30 seconds of work / 15 seconds of rest
Equipment: mat, optional weights

Round 1
Reverse lunge with press
Walking side squats
Curtsy lunge to right with double bicep curl
Curtsy lunge to left with double bicep curl
Jumping jacks
*Repeat round 1 only

Round 2
Russian twists
Single bent-knee leg drops
Reach-throughs
Low plank hip dips

Round 3
Bridges
Sweep-throughs on all fours, right
Sweep-throughs on all fours, left
Fire hydrants, right
Fire hydrants, left
Body weight tricep dips

Round 4
Narrow squat with a pulse
Skater hops
Side lunge knee to chest, right
Side lunge knee to chest, left

Round 5
Arms to the side, bent elbows, and pulse
Arms in front, bent elbows, and pulse
Arm scissors
45-degree arm backward pulses

Round 6
Deadlifts
Plie calf raises

Round 7
Russian twists
Single bent-knee leg drops
Reach-throughs
Low plank hip dips

Round 8
Bridges
Sweep-throughs on all fours, right
Sweep-throughs on all fours, left
Fire hydrants, right
Fire hydrants, left

Food

Breakfast: Blueberry Greek Yogurt Pancakes (page 237)

Morning Snack

Lunch: Mango Shrimp Tacos (page 254)

Afternoon Snack

Dinner: Halibut and Veggie Skewers (page 281)

Evening Protein Snack

Daily Task

Meal Prep. The one task for today is to tackle your first day of meal prep, and then schedule the remaining meal prep days in your calendar. Intimidated by cooking several recipes at once? Turn to page 285 for some tips and tricks to make it easier.

Day 2

Everyone can get to day 2, right? Not always. Congratulations on stepping into the next twenty-four hours. It's an ab-tastic kind of day today with a glute burn added into the mix!

> If you made it once, you can make it again. Imagine the view from the top.

Workout: Six-Pack Abs and Perky Butt

Circuit workout: Do each round twice before moving to the next round.

45 seconds of work / 15 seconds of rest
Equipment: mat

Round 1
Narrow deadlifts
Walking side squats
Bicycles
Flutter kicks

Round 2
Bridges with pulse to side at the top
Walking in-and-out bridges
Plank dips
Dead bugs with opposite arm and leg extension

Round 3
Single-leg Romanian deadlifts, right
Single-leg Romanian deadlifts, left
Full sit-up
Opposite-elbow mountain climbers

Round 4
Squat jumps
High plank

Food

Breakfast: Reboot Spinach and Almond Butter Smoothie (page 235)

Morning Snack

Lunch: Veggie Lover's Chili (page 260)

Afternoon Snack

Dinner: Blueberry Balsamic Turkey Meatballs (page 266)

Evening Snack

Daily Task

Tonight, before you go to bed, plan out your day ahead. Get organized and schedule in all the things that you want to accomplish. Be specific with your timing. You will realize you have a lot more time and the minutes seem longer when you plan like this. From the moment you wake up to when you are going to bed, know what you are going to do!

Day 3

You are basically halfway through your first week once you complete this day. Boom! How does that make you feel? Creating healthy habits just means putting your best foot forward each day, following the plan, and always visualizing the results you are going to get from being consistent. Ready to see that sweat?

> "You can't change your destination overnight; you can change your direction." —Jim Rohn

Workout: Kickboxing Cardio

*30 seconds of exercise / 10 seconds of rest. Once through, then start from the top until the *.*
Equipment: mat

Front punches
Side shuffle across mat
Kick to right
Kick to left
Pull down "Yes," right
Pull down "Yes," left
Undercut, right
Undercut, left
Side shuffle undercut and punch forward, right, and side kick
Side shuffle undercut and punch forward, left, and side kick

Squat kick to the back, right hook
Squat kick to the back, left hook
Knee to chest, right
Knee to chest, left
Kick forward and curtsy lunge, right
Kick forward and curtsy lunge, left
*
Knee to chest, punch forward, undercut, and kick to side, right
Knee to chest, punch forward, undercut, and kick to side, left
Wide squat quick feet
Punches in V-sit
Bicycles
Frog jumps with double punch
Alternate side kicks

Food

Breakfast: Sweet Potato Toast with Avocado and Egg (page 241)
Morning Snack
Lunch: Pesto Tuna Wrap (page 250)
Afternoon Snack
Dinner: Teriyaki Tuna with Roasted Green Beans and Soba (page 273)
Evening Protein Snack

Daily Task

Start journaling. Write our your feelings, your morning affirmations, and the great events of the day! Add in five things for which you are grateful for that day. It could be a person or something you have in your life—or just the fact you have the ability to move. Start making this a daily habit and it will soon put life into perspective and you'll be looking at the glass half full.

Day 4

How did we get to day 4 already? It's flying by because you are keeping full and getting in the best burn on the planet. Yes, I might be biased about my workouts. Or you might be thinking, "Holy shit, is it only day 4—how am I going to keep going?" The great news is that you *can* keep going because the first step in success is *choice*. Pull those big-girl pants on and let's keep going! I am right here behind you to give a gentle kick to the backside. Let's get sweaty with some cardio!

> Surround yourself with almond butter, not negativity.

Workout: Targeted Lower Body

Stacked workouts: 1st and 2nd exercise; 1st, 2nd, and 3rd exercise; 1st, 2nd, 3rd, and 4th exercise; and so on. Rounds 1 and 2 are separate.

30 seconds of exercise / 15 seconds of rest
Equipment: mat, optional weights

Round 1
Squat to heel raise to reach up
Lateral step to squat
Alternating curtsy lunge with pulses
Deadlift to squat

Round 1 (continued)
Alternating fire hydrants
Static bridge hold

Round 2
Alternating single deadlift taking 3 steps back
Goblet squat
Skater hops
Alternating reverse lunge with pulse
Wide plie calf raises
Alternating standing leg lifts

Food

Breakfast: Blueberry Greek Yogurt Pancakes (page 237)
Morning Snack
Lunch: Mango Shrimp Tacos (page 254)
Afternoon Snack
Dinner: Halibut and Veggie Skewers (page 281)
Evening Protein Snack

Daily Task

Do a quick clear-out to release some weight off your shoulders. Delete old texts, unopened emails, and voicemails. There's nothing worse than looking at your phone with a bunch of red notifications everywhere! Clear it out. You might also need to have another rummage in your pantry, to clean out some items that were not on your shopping list. You could even throw out a person whom you would be better off not having in your life. Declutter, feel lighter, and make room for the new.

Day 5

We sure did sweat yesterday in our lower-body workout, and I am proud of you. I would not be surprised if you hate me during the workout—you might even swear and curse at me! That's okay, as I know the results are coming and one day you will meet me and say, "Look, Rebecca—feel my abs!" as you grab my hand to place on your belly! Just remember that the burn is temporary, because you are going to need that in your head through today's workout. I'm so excited for it, so grab those bands and let's go!

> If you still look cute after the gym, then you didn't work out hard enough!

Workout: Toned Upper Body

Circuit workout: Do each round twice before moving to the next round.

30 seconds of exercise / 15 seconds of rest
Equipment: mat, optional resistance bands and weights

Round 1
Arms to the side, bent elbows, and pulse
Arms in front, bent elbows, and pulse
Hold a squat, palms in front, pulses
Flys

Round 2
Kneeling bicep curl
Plank shoulder taps
Body weight tricep dip taps
Superman arms in front pulses

Round 3
Squeeze elbow to waist
Overhead pull-downs
Arm scissors
Arms out to side, palms back, pulse
Arms out to side, palms front, pulse

Round 4
Rows
Overhead press
Lying-down chest press
Lying-down chest pulses

Round 5
Wide push-ups
Elbows out circle backward
Elbows out circle forward

Food

Breakfast: Parmesan Veggie Frittata (page 239)

Morning Snack

Lunch: Pesto Tuna Wrap (page 250)

Afternoon Snack

Dinner: Lemon-Herb Chicken Pasta (page 270)
Evening Protein Snack

Daily Task

Pose naked in front of the mirror. Yep, that's right—take off all your clothes and stand butt-naked in front of the mirror. Add in your daily affirmations here, too—why not, let's go for it. Look at yourself and be like, "Darn, you just did five days of being a badass." Shake it, touch it, and look at it. You are giving your body good nutrition and exercise and feeding your mind positive stuff. Be proud and say, "Body, I am doing this for us!"

Day 6

Okay, let's just take a moment, because we are pretty cool. Yep, I told you that you're cool, so it's basically a fact. I was definitely not cool at school—far from it, in fact. I would sit with my best friend twenty feet from where the cool gang was, so we felt like we were basically part of it. This is why I created my own cool gang, and you are officially invited to join! My door always stays open. It's also pretty cool that it's day 6, which means you're only one day away from crushing your first week. If you did your best, that's all that matters. Don't let yourself down today, because we need to work out those obliques!

> When you feel like quitting,
> remember why you started.

Workout: Obliques Burn

30 seconds of work / 15 seconds of rest

Equipment: mat, optional weights

Alternating side planks
Oblique crunches on your side, right
Oblique crunches on your side, left
Low plank hip dips

Slow bicycles
Side plank with hip dips, right
Side plank with hip dips, left
Russian twist

Opposite toe touches
Star touches
Kneeling crescent moon pulses, right
Kneeling crescent moon pulses, left

Knee-to-elbow taps
Leg drops on diagonal
Full sit-up twist to right, pulse
Full sit-up twist to left, pulse

Across-the-body mountain climbers
Bicycles with 3 pulses on each side
Dead bugs, right elbow to touch knee
Dead bugs, left elbow to touch knee

Alternating heel touches
Full sit-up with Russian twist at top
Running man bicycles
Alternating side plank reach-throughs

Reverse knee-to-elbow taps

Food

Breakfast: Sweet Potato Toast with Avocado and Egg (page 241)
Morning Snack
Lunch: Grilled Chicken and Peach Salad (page 256)
Afternoon Snack
Dinner: Teriyaki Tuna with Roasted Green Beans and Soba (page 273)
Evening Protein Snack

Daily Task

Set your new personal goal and start it. There is something on the tip of your tongue, the forefront of your mind, the front of your shoe—so what exactly is stopping you from getting it out? Whatever the roadblock, today is the day to let it go and get started on what you really want to do. It doesn't matter how big or small you think it is; just do it!

Day 7

Woo-hoo, we made it to day 7, the first week, a new milestone! Let's celebrate! You know you can do it, and even if you weren't 100 percent successful, it doesn't matter! You went for it and you're creating those good habits, so let's work together to finish the coming weeks strong. Your life is a big collection of days, so stop complaining. It's just thirty days of your life. Let's go!

When I lost all of my excuses, I found my results.

Workout: De-Stress

Hold each stretch for 40 seconds and go through twice.
Equipment: mat

Child's pose
Cobra
Downward-facing dog
Seated twists, right
Seated twists, left
Kneeling side oblique stretch, right
Kneeling side oblique stretch, left
Lying down, extend arms and legs in opposite direction
Knee to chest

Supine twist, right
Supine twist, left
Happy baby pose
Heart opener
Standing forward fold
Eagle pose, right
Eagle pose, left
Pigeon pose, right
Pigeon pose, left

Food

Breakfast: Parmesan Veggie Frittata (page 239)
Morning Snack
Lunch: Veggie Lover's Chili (page 260)
Afternoon Snack
Dinner: Blueberry Balsamic Turkey Meatballs (page 266)
Evening Protein Snack

Daily Task

Instead of thinking, just do! 5, 4, 3, 2, 1 . . . and we are off. Practice this today whenever you need it. Wake up, get your workout in, stick to your meal plan. Check out all the amazing tools you are learning that are going to shape you into being healthier and happier so you can go after your biggest dreams!

DAYS 8–15

Shopping List

Dairy and Protein

Chicken breast, boneless and skinless (½ pound)
Cod (two 4-ounce fillets)
Eggs (1 dozen)
Feta (1 container, if needed)
Mozzarella, shredded (1 small bag)
Smoked salmon (2 ounces)
Tofu (two two 16-ounce containers, one firm, one extra-firm)
Turkey, ground 99% lean (1½ pounds)

Produce

Apple, Granny Smith (2)
Arugula (1 large container)
Asparagus (1 bunch)
Avocados (2)
Baby spinach (one 5-ounce package)
Banana (1)
Bell peppers, red (1) and yellow (2)
Blueberries (one 4.4-ounce container)
Broccoli slaw (1 bag)
Butternut squash, peeled and cubed (2 cups)
Button mushrooms (one 10-ounce package)
Cauliflower (2 heads)
Coleslaw mix, no dressing (1 bag)
Celery (1 small bunch)
Cucumber, English (1)
Ginger, fresh (1 large "hand")
Grapes, red seedless (½ cup)
Grape tomatoes (1 container)
Green beans (10 ounces)
Herbs, fresh: basil (1 large bunch), cilantro (1 bunch), dill (1 small container), mint (1 small container)
Kale (1 small bunch)
Kiwi (1)
Limes (4)
Mango (1)

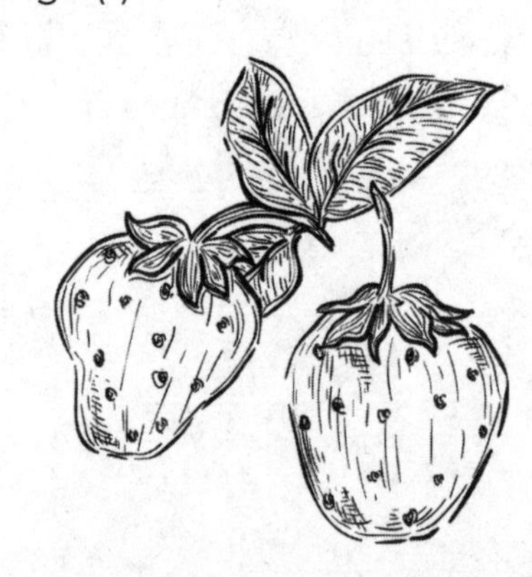

Mung bean sprouts (1 cup)
Onion, red (1 small)
Orange (1)
Scallions (1 bunch)
Spaghetti squash, small (1)
Strawberries (1 small container)
Sweet potato (1)
Zucchini (1)

Other

Bread: sliced whole wheat bread (use 1 slice, freeze remainder))

Meal Prep Plan

Day 8: Before you begin, prepare 3 hard-boiled eggs (plus more for snacks) and 1 cup quinoa. Prepare California Veggie Bowl (all in fridge), Greek Power Bowl with Shrimp (in fridge), Veggie Pizza with Cauliflower Crust (1 crust and sauce portion in fridge/1 crust and sauce portion in freezer), Berry Breakfast Pops, Greek Turkey Burgers (all in fridge), and Tofu Veggie Scramble (all in fridge).

Day 12: Prepare Sweet Tofu and Cauliflower Salad (all in fridge), No-Bake Lime Coconut Protein Bites (2 portions in fridge/3 in freezer), Turkey and Kale Breakfast Bake (2 portions in fridge/4 in freezer), Turkey Egg Roll in a Bowl (1 portion in fridge/2 in freezer), Light Tofu Thai Curry (2 portions in fridge/1 in freezer), and Mango Shrimp Tacos (all in fridge).

Fresh Prep: If possible, prepare these meals when you are ready to eat them: Smoked Salmon Avocado Toast, and Spaghetti Squash with Tomato Sauce and Cod (refrigerate the second portion).

Plan your snacks: Choose what appeals to you from the list on pages 140–141, planning for three per day.

Day 8

Once this week is done, you're halfway there! Variety is the spice of life, which is why today we are trying something a little new. My ballet workouts are some of my most popular because we get to dance through the burn! And today that burn is for your booty. It's time to feel like a badass ballerina!

> If you aren't willing to work hard for it, then don't complain about not having it.

Workout: Ballet Burn Bootcamp

Stacked workouts: 1st and 2nd exercise; 1st, 2nd, and 3rd exercise; 1st, 2nd, 3rd, and 4th exercise; and so on. Rounds 1 and 2 are separate.

30 seconds of work / 15 seconds of rest
Equipment: mat, optional weights

Round 1
Wide plie squat
Alternating side leg extensions, 3 lifts
Slow plie in first position
Plie and alternating backward leg lift
Plie jumps
Second-position heel raises

Round 2
Alternating leg lift with circles
First- to second-position arms
Calf raise to side leg extensions
Small steps, feet together on balls of feet
Wide plie pulses
Alternating forward lunge

Food

Breakfast: Smoked Salmon Avocado Toast (page 236)
Morning Snack
Lunch: California Veggie Bowl (page 262)
Afternoon Snack
Dinner: Lemon-Herb Chicken Pasta (page 270)
Evening Protein Snack

Daily Task

Get up earlier. It's amazing what you can do with just an extra thirty minutes in the morning. Set your alarm tomorrow for thirty minutes earlier (which means going to bed a little earlier, too), and give yourself a little more time to get ready, eat breakfast, read, and prepare to have a kick-ass day!

Day 9

There will be days when you can't wait to work out, and there will be days when it is the last thing you want to do. Once you've committed and you have done it, you'll be so glad you made the effort. Nothing like getting a little bit (or a lot) of sweat in your life!

Which wine pairs well with squats?

Workout: Back, Chest, and Shoulders

30 seconds of work / 15 seconds of rest. Once through, then start from the bottom and work back to the top of the list.
Equipment: mat, weights

Upright row
Front arm extensions
Overhead press, elbows in
Flys with row

Narrow push-ups
Overhead tricep dips
V-extensions
Superwoman extension
Superman, elbows to waist

Wide push-ups
Chest press
Inner chest press
Bent-over row, right
Bent-over row, left
Hammer curl

Arm pulses to the side, palms up
Arm pulses to the side, palms down
Arm pulses forward, palms facing together
Arm pulses forward, palms facing apart
Front punches

Upright row
Front arm extensions
Overhead press, elbows in
Flys with row

Narrow push-ups
Overhead tricep dips
V-extensions
Superwoman extension
Superman, elbows to waist

Wide push-ups
Chest press
Inner chest press
Bent-over row, right
Bent-over row, left
Hammer curl

Food

Breakfast: Berry Breakfast Pop (page 246)

Morning Snack

Lunch: Greek Power Bowl with Shrimp (page 264)

Afternoon Snack

Dinner: Veggie Pizza with Cauliflower Crust (page 275)

Evening Protein Snack

Daily Task

When was the last time you increased your weights? Well, if you haven't in the last four weeks, now is the time! Push yourself and see what you can do—you won't get bulky, and it will snap you out of a plateau.

Day 10

Yesterday's task was to increase the weights, and there is nothing better than lifting heavy when you are doing glutes, which is what I have on the menu for you today! I love to mix cardio and strength training; to pair with our glute exercises, we are going to add in cardio. We are a third of the way there. Ask yourself if you are giving it all you have. Could you do better?

> You either suffer the pain of discipline
> or you suffer the pain of regret.

Workout: Cardio and Butt Build

Stacked workouts: 1st and 2nd exercise; 1st, 2nd, and 3rd exercise; 1st, 2nd, 3rd, and 4th exercise; and so on. Rounds 1 and 2 are separate.

30 seconds of work / 15 seconds of rest
Equipment: mat, weights

Round 1
Forward lunge to 3 backward leg lifts
Skater hops
Single leg deadlift, 3 on each side
Jump in and out
Bridge hold on heels
On knees, alternating single leg extensions backward

Round 2
Curtsy lunge with kick
Narrow deadlift
Alternating fire hydrants with diagonal kick
Alternating single-leg bridges
Stand up, kneel down
Squat jumps

Food

Breakfast: Blueberry Greek Yogurt Pancakes (page 237)
Morning Snack
Lunch: Veggie Lover's Chili (page 260)
Afternoon Snack
Dinner: Spaghetti Squash with Tomato Sauce and Cod (page 277)
Evening Protein Snack

Daily Task

Go through your bank statements. It might seem tiresome, yet you will be thanking me when you save money each month. There could be a few items coming out of your account that you don't even know about, or maybe you're spending more on items than you should, so it's a great practice to routinely check your account. Reviewing your statements will also help you avoid overdraft fees and make you aware of your spending and saving habits.

Day 11

How long does it take to create a habit and make it part of your routine? Well, that depends on you. Everyone is different, so instead of thinking, "Okay, if I do this for twenty-one days it will become a habit," say to yourself, "I will do this for as long as it takes until it becomes a habit." If after twenty-one days it isn't coming naturally to you, that doesn't matter, because you are on your own journey. Right! Let's keep on forming that fitness habit and tone up the upper body!

> The real workout starts when you feel like quitting.

Workout: Strong and Lean Upper Body

Circuit workout: Do each round twice before moving to the next round.

45 seconds of work / 15 seconds of rest
Equipment: mat, weights

Round 1
Tricep kickback and overhead press
Compass jacks
High plank and arm lift to side
Single rows and double row

Round 2
Thumbs-up back lifts
Squat to single-arm press
Isometric V-sit
Two front punches with a fly

Round 3
Palms face forward and pulse
Bicep curl halfway
Dead bugs with alternating leg extensions
Frog jumps

Round 4
Hammer curl to diagonal arm extension
High plank to low plank

Food

Breakfast: Tofu Veggie Scramble (page 243)

Morning Snack

Lunch: California Veggie Bowl (page 262)

Afternoon Snack

Dinner: Greek Turkey Burger (page 268)

Evening Protein Snack

Daily Task

Write down your new morning routine. You've read about it, and today we are going to put pen to paper and create yours. Writing gets your brain to connect and take ownership and responsibility. Map out your morning routine in fifteen-minute increments (turn to pages 130–132 if you need a refresher).

Day 12

Today we are going to use one of my favorite pieces of equipment: the resistance band. I love these because they really take your workout to the next level, get you feeling the burn, and are easy to carry around with you. You do not have to use them in this workout, though I recommend that you try them and challenge yourself! Check out the Burn Bands at the Rebecca-Louise.com shop to really feel the part!

Take the risk or lose the chance.

Workout: Total Body Tone

*45 seconds of work / 15 seconds of rest. Once through, then start from the top until the *.*
Equipment: mat, optional weights and resistance bands

Hold a squat with front arm pulses
Twisting lunges
Plank jumps
Overhead sit-up
Knees to chest and extend
Single-leg lunges, right
Single-leg lunges, left
Tricep dips, touch opposite legs
Inchworms

Low leg circles, right
Low leg circles, left
*
Fly with pulses
Repeaters, right
Repeaters, left

Food

Breakfast: Turkey and Kale Breakfast Bake (page 247)
Morning Snack
Lunch: Sweet Tofu and Cauliflower Salad (page 258)
Afternoon Snack
Dinner: Spaghetti Squash with Tomato Sauce and Cod (page 277)
Evening Protein Snack

Daily Task

Put on your favorite song and dance to it. Yes, you read this right! We have talked about changing our state of mind and getting ourselves out of a funk. So, whether you're feeling chipper or you're in a grumpy mood, today's task is going to get you vibrating at a whole new level. What is that song of yours that when you play it all your troubles seem to fade away? Put it on as loud as it will go and dance like nobody's watching. You will be smiling from ear to ear. Once you have given this a shot today, you will start to use it more often. Come on, don't be shy—you've got this!

Day 13

Hopefully you're tired from last night's dance party! Next up we are going to fight out all that frustration and be badass warriors. When you feel like you need a break, the best way forward is to move your body. Exercise will increase your adrenaline and give you a good buzz, one without drinking booze! Get focused for today's workout, during which you can let it all out.

> Some days I amaze myself; other days I put my keys in the fridge.

Workout: Body Combat

30 seconds of exercise / 15 seconds of rest. Go through twice.
Equipment: mat

Exercise
Punches to diagonal right
Punches to diagonal left
Squat with fists to chin
Alternating undercuts

Exercise
Repeaters, right
Repeaters, left
Quick feet for 3 seconds and jog for 3 seconds

Hook right and squat
Hook left and squat
Kick forward and lunge back, right
Kick forward and lunge back, left

Punches forward
Kick to the right side and punch forward
Kick to the left side and punch forward
Squat in and out

Alternating knee to chest and kick to side
Kick to side and side lunge, right
Kick to side and side lunge, left
Side shuffle across mat

Two punches, two undercuts, and side kick, right
Two punches, two undercuts, and side kick, left
Single knee lifts, right
Single knee lifts, left
Sit-up and 2 front punches

Leg drops to punch upward
Bridge with chest press
Sit-up and 2 front punches
Leg drop, sit-up to punch upward

Punches to diagonal right
Punches to diagonal left
Squat with fists to chin
Alternating undercuts
Repeaters, right
Repeaters, left

Food

Breakfast: No-Bake Lime Coconut Protein Bites (page 249)
Morning Snack
Lunch: Mango Shrimp Tacos (page 254)
Afternoon Snack
Dinner: Light Tofu Thai Curry (page 279)
Evening Protein Snack

Daily Task

Look back at all your accomplishments. So often we are so focused on the future, thinking about what our next goal is and beating ourselves up for not being there yet. Spend at least thirty minutes today looking back at your life and writing all the things you've accomplished. How have you made yourself proud? It could be passing a test, getting a new job, that time you took flowers to a friend, or simply opening the door for someone when you were in a hurry. Seeing all the amazing things you've already done will give you the confidence to keep going.

Day 14

Today you have woken up realizing how amazing you are and all the things you have accomplished. It's important each week to give your body time to recover and repair, so today we have a set of great exercises to get you energized! You might think that these "easy days" are the ones you can skip, when in fact they are the most important. Your body and mind deserve it.

> Watch your thoughts; they become words.
> Watch your words; they become actions.
> Watch your actions; they become habits.
> Watch your habits; they become character.
> Watch your character; it becomes your destiny.

Workout: Energizing Stretch

Hold each stretch for 45 seconds.
Equipment: mat

Cat and cow
Runner's lunge, right
Runner's lunge, left
Runner's lunge with twists, right
Runner's lunge with twists, left
Pigeon pose, right

Pigeon pose, left
Frog pose
Warrior 1, right
Warrior 1, left
Kneeling oblique stretch, right
Kneeling oblique stretch, left
Seated forward fold
Calf stretch, right
Calf stretch, left
Walking toe touches
Standing knee hugs, right
Standing knee hugs, left
Mountain pose, stretching your arms above your head
Tree pose, right
Tree pose, left
Cat and cow
Runner's lunge, right
Runner's lunge, left
Runner's lunge with twists, right
Runner's lunge with twists, left
Pigeon pose, right
Pigeon pose, left

Food

Breakfast: Tofu Veggie Scramble (page 243)

Morning Snack

Lunch: Turkey Egg Roll in a Bowl (page 252)

Afternoon Snack

Dinner: Greek Turkey Burger (page 268)

Evening Protein Snack

Daily Task

Set a new business goal. Even if you don't think that you are business minded, I know that you have goals and ideas you want to see come to life. It doesn't matter whether this idea is about making money or not—the objective is to get you to dream and have some fun being creative. Once you've set this goal, the next twenty-four hours are going to be crucial in taking action. So what is the first step you need to do to take this from paper to reality? Make that step, then keep adding steps along this journey.

Day 15

Just like that, we are halfway through our thirty days together! You see, it really was as much fun as I promised! Remember to get the first step of yesterday's business goal into action—whatever you do, just do something. And if you haven't quite got the confidence to do it yet, tackle today's workout to get that adrenaline pumping through your body!

> The secret of your future is hidden in your daily routine.

Workout: Ab Attack

30 seconds of work / 15 seconds of rest. Do each exercise 2 times and move to the next.
Equipment: mat

Plank forward and backward
Single leg drops
Slow sit-ups
Bird dog
Low plank hold
Crunches
Flutter kicks at 45 degrees
Straight-up toe touches

Low plank hold
Side crunches, right
Side crunches, left
V-sit hold
Low plank dips
On all fours, lift your knees off the ground
Starfish sit-ups
V-sit crunch
Reach-throughs
Dead bug static hold
Full sit-up, legs straight
Double leg drops
Bird dog with a pulse
Straight bicycles
Mountain climbers
Hold legs at 45 degrees

Plank forward and backward
Single leg drops
Slow sit-ups
Bird dog
Low plank hold
Crunches
Flutter kicks at 45 degrees
Straight-up toe touches
Low plank hold
Side crunches, right
Side crunches, left
V-sit hold
Low plank dips

Food

Breakfast: Turkey and Kale Breakfast Bake (page 247)
Morning Snack
Lunch: Mango Shrimp Tacos (page 254)
Afternoon Snack
Dinner: Light Tofu Thai Curry (page 279)
Evening Protein Snack

Daily Task

Disconnect from your phone for the evening. Technology often leaves us confused as to what the "real world" really is—we're so caught up in our electronics! Even watching TV can put us into another world where we are immersed in something that is not our own reality. Put the phone away, turn off your laptop and TV, and connect with your partner, friends, and family, giving them all your attention and focus. If you live on your own, give that time to yourself. It might even be a little uncomfortable at the beginning as you navigate relationships without distractions. This is how you get to a deeper and more meaningful connection that is more important than anything going on in your phone.

DAYS 16–22

Shopping List

Dairy and Protein

Chicken breast, boneless and skinless (½ pound)
Eggs, large (½ dozen)
Feta (1 container)
Fish and seafood: cod (two 4-ounce fillets), salmon (one 3-ounce fillet; two 4-ounce fillets, skin on), tuna (two 4-ounce steaks), shrimp (fresh, 10 ounces), shrimp (frozen, peeled, and deveined, medium (one 1-pound bag))
Parmesan cheese (if needed)
Smoked salmon (2 ounces)

Produce

Arugula (1 small container or bunch)
Asparagus (1 bunch)
Avocado (2)
Baby spinach (one 5-ounce container)
Banana (1)
Bell pepper, yellow (1)
Broccoli (1 head or 4 cups florets)
Fingerling potatoes (6 ounces)
Grape tomatoes (one 10-ounce container)
Green beans (6 ounces)
Lemon (1)
Limes (2)
Mango (1)
Onion, red (1 small)
Peaches, small (2)
Scallions (1 bunch)
Spaghetti squash, small (1)
Sweet potato (2)
Zoodles (zucchini noodles, 1 package, or 2 large zucchini)
Zucchini (1)

Other

Soba noodles (1 bundle)

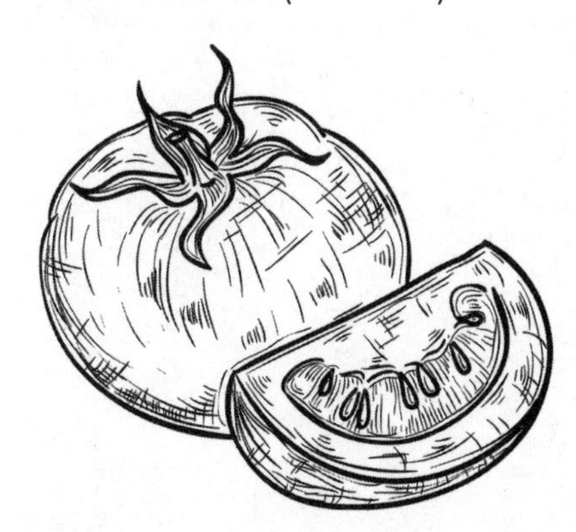

Meal Prep Plan

Day 16: Before you begin, prepare 2 hard-boiled eggs (plus more for snacks) and 1 cup quinoa. Prepare Sheet Pan Shrimp and Broccoli (dinner tonight/second portion in fridge), Sweet Potato Toast with Avocado and Egg (all in fridge), and Feta and Spinach Salmon Salad (in fridge). Grill chicken for Grilled Chicken and Peach Salad (in fridge).

Day 19: Prepare Teriyaki Tuna with Roasted Green Beans and Soba (all in fridge), Mango Shrimp Tacos (all in fridge), and California Veggie Bowl (all in fridge).

Fresh prep: If possible, prepare these when you're ready to enjoy them: Reboot Spinach and Almond Butter Smoothie, Spaghetti Squash with Tomato Sauce and Cod (refrigerate the second portion), Smoked Salmon Avocado Toast, Lemon Parmesan Salmon Zoodles (refrigerate the second portion).

Plan your snacks: Choose what appeals to you from the list on pages 140–141, planning for three per day.

Day 16

One of my favorite workouts is coming up today, and I challenge you to increase your weights if you've been using the same ones for a month or longer. It's time to prove to yourself that you can do more than what you first thought when you woke up this morning, both mentally and physically. Let's pick stuff up and put it down!

> Action is what gets you started.
> Habit is what keeps you going.

Workout: Head-to-Toe Heavy Weights

Stacked workouts: 1st and 2nd exercise; 1st, 2nd, and 3rd exercise; 1st, 2nd, 3rd, and 4th exercise; and so on. Rounds 1 and 2 are separate.

30 seconds of work / 15 seconds of rest
Equipment: mat, weights

Round 1
Alternating curtsy lunges with a pulse
Bicep curl to overhead press
Alternating forward lunges with hammer curl
Alternating side planks with arm extensions
Squat to snatch
Hip thrusts with knee pulse

Round 2
Narrow squats to side tap
Deadlift to rows
Stand up, squat pulse, and down to knees
Fly to tricep extension
Weighted calf raises
Flutter kicks

Food

Breakfast: Berry Breakfast Pop (page 246)
Morning Snack
Lunch: Sweet Tofu and Cauliflower Salad (page 258)
Afternoon Snack
Dinner: Sheet Pan Shrimp and Broccoli (page 272)
Evening Protein Snack

Daily Task

Embrace your evening routine. Unwinding from the day is just as important as setting up the day. This is the time you can focus on self-care and really take a moment for yourself, which will help you sleep better and feel rested for the next day ahead. Enjoy a longer shower, take a bath, or spend time washing your face and putting on night cream. Read a book while sipping on some calming tea and give yourself ten to fifteen minutes to stretch. Start this process ninety minutes before you hit the pillow to allow yourself not to be rushed. You will thank me for it in the morning.

Day 17

Being well rested and raring to go after a great night's sleep is just what you needed, because today we are about to turn it up, bust out a whole bunch of cardio moves, and get sweaty! I love to mix up the workouts from weights to cardio to yoga and more. This way your body improves its strength, flexibility, and endurance—all areas to focus on when building overall fitness and health.

> Exercise in the morning . . . before your brain figures out what you're doing.

Workout: Fire Me Up Cardio

Circuit workout: Do each round twice before moving to the next round.

30 seconds of work / 15 seconds of rest
Equipment: mat

Round 1
Booty kickers
Alternating side lunge
Mountain climbers
Side shuffles
Slow squats

Round 2
Frog jumps
High knees
Star jumps
Squat side kicks
Taps to side

Round 3
Bicycles
Side steps to tuck jump
Burpees
Squat jumps
Calf raises

Food

Breakfast: Reboot Spinach and Almond Butter Smoothie (page 235)

Morning Snack

Lunch: Feta and Spinach Salmon Salad (page 265)

Afternoon Snack

Dinner: Spaghetti Squash with Tomato Sauce and Cod (page 277)

Evening Protein Snack

Daily Task

Send three voice messages. Saying something nice to someone makes for a deeper connection. Although you can do it through words in a text message, there is nothing like the sound of your voice. People can hear the passion and authenticity when you are speaking as well as feel your words. Today send out three voice messages to people and tell them what they mean to you. I promise you, this will make someone's day.

Day 18

I hope you have woken up to a couple of nice replies to your voice messages this morning and you are feeling and receiving love. It's amazing how your mood can change by the simple act of giving. Today is no different: You're going to give love to your upper body, focusing on the chest and arms. Let's start the pump!

> "Look after your body;
> it's the only place you have to live."
> —Jim Rohn

Workout: Strengthen Upper Body and Tone Arms

30 seconds of work / 15 seconds of rest.
Equipment: mat, weights

Elbows-out pulls
Overhead press with pulse
Tricep overhead extensions
Flys
Forward arm extensions
In-and-out shoulder
Push-ups
High-to-low plank

Lying-down chest press
Superwoman's hold
Single-arm press, right
Single-arm press, left
Superwoman, bring elbows to waist and extend forward
Alternating plank rows
Lateral arm extensions

Lying-down narrow chest press
Bicep curls with in-and-out pulse
Hammer curls
Mountain climbers
Side plank reach-throughs, right
Side plank reach-throughs, left
Inchworms
Diagonal punches
Arnolds

Elbows-out pulls
Overhead press with pulse
Tricep overhead extensions
Flys
Forward arm extensions
In-and-out shoulder
Push-ups
High-to-low plank
Lying-down chest press
Superwoman's hold
Single-arm press, right
Single-arm press, left
Superwoman, bring elbows to waist and extend forward
Alternating plank rows
Lateral arm extensions

Food

Breakfast: No-Bake Lime Coconut Protein Bites (page 249)
Morning Snack
Lunch: Grilled Chicken and Peach Salad (page 256)
Afternoon Snack
Dinner: Sheet Pan Shrimp and Broccoli (page 272)
Evening Protein Snack

Daily Task

Book a trip. Yes, right now. Get something in your diary for a trip within the next month with your partner, friends, or family, or go solo. It could be that you go to a park or the beach, or you could have an overnight stay somewhere. You can make it whatever you like; just get something scheduled today that will set the intention to go have fun, explore, and mix up your scenery. Schedule your fun first—you are never too busy to live your best life!

Day 19

Take note of how your body is feeling today. Are you feeling more energized or are you tired? Either way, it's exactly how you are meant to feel. Just because you are starting a challenge and expecting to feel a certain way, this doesn't always happen. If you are feeling a little tired because you are not used to doing this much exercise, that's okay. You still want to move your body each day; just drop the intensity down a little. Feeding your body the right nutrition is going to be essential for keeping you fueled!

> You can't have a million-dollar dream with a minimum-wage work effort.

Workout: Lower Body Tone

40 seconds of work / 15 seconds of rest.
Equipment: mat, optional weights and resistance bands

Alternating standing leg extensions to side with a squat
Wide deadlifts
Bridge, alternating single knee to chest
Lying down side leg lifts, right
Lying down side leg lifts, left
Fire hydrants, right
Fire hydrants, left

Jump in and outs
Goblet squat
Lunge to 3 leg lifts, right
Lunge to 3 leg lifts, left
Alternating reverse leg extension with squat
Reverse lunge, bring knee to chest, right
Reverse lunge, bring knee to chest, left
Low squat pulses
Side lunge with pulses, right
Side lunge with pulses, left
Standing leg lifts, knee to chest, right
Standing leg lifts, knee to chest, left
Narrow deadlift with steps to back

Narrow deadlift with steps to back
Standing leg lifts, knee to chest, left
Standing leg lifts, knee to chest, right
Side lunge with pulses, left
Side lunge with pulses, right
Low squat pulses
Reverse lunge, bring knee to chest, left
Reverse lunge, bring knee to chest, right
Alternating reverse leg extension with squat

Food

Breakfast: Turkey and Kale Breakfast Bake (page 247)

Morning Snack

Lunch: Veggie Lover's Chili (page 260)

Afternoon Snack

Dinner: Veggie Pizza with Cauliflower Crust (page 275)

Evening Protein Snack

Daily Task

Who is in your circle of influence? Today is the big day, the day to clear out your friends list of people who might not be serving you to your highest purpose. Write down the five people you hang around with the most. Now, looking at this list, do you aspire to be like them or look up to them? You might look up to one or two of them, or you may realize that you aspire to be like none of them. This is your opportunity to get real with yourself and figure out what it is you want out of life and if you are going to level up. Leveling up starts with your environment, and today is the day you choose with whom you are going to spend most of your time.

Day 20

We are clearing out all the things that are taking up unwanted space to allow room for all the new things that are going to bring more positivity and joy to your life and get you the results you want. It's time for some Pilates today—we're going to get a great stretch and strengthen your core.

> Your life isn't yours if you constantly care what other people think.

Workout: Pilates Power

Circuit workout: Do each round twice before moving to the next round.

30 seconds of work / 15 seconds of rest
Equipment: mat

Round 1
Low plank
Bridge, bring hands under
Single-leg bridges, right
Single-leg bridges, left
Windmills

Round 2
Scissors
V-sit hold
High plank heel raises
Opposite toe touches
Starfish hold

Round 3
Plie squats
Plie heel raises
Bridge hold
Bicycles
Twist upper body and touch opposite toes, right
Twist upper body and touch opposite toes, left

Round 4
Tricep dips
Wide scissors, grab each leg
Downward dog leg extensions
Alternating side plank crunch

Food

Breakfast: Smoked Salmon Avocado Toast (page 236)

Morning Snack

Lunch: Mango Shrimp Tacos (page 254)

Afternoon Snack

Dinner: Spaghetti Squash with Tomato Sauce and Cod (page 277)

Evening Protein Snack

Daily Task

While you're on a roll with "out with the old, in with the new," we are going to attack your closet today. If you have lost weight and still have clothes that you used to wear, they can't be in your possession a minute longer. Part of the process of growing into your new identity is letting go of the past. Donate old clothing that you have not worn for more than a year (I mean, we do have seasons, so remember, spring comes around again!) or any clothes that do not fit you. Let go physically so you can then let go emotionally.

Day 21

I have a treat for you today with the best stretches to help with back stiffness and soreness. We spend so much time looking down at our phones or laptops that it is changing the shape of our frames and causing issues later on in life. We get to spend today relieving some of that tension and feeling a little lighter.

I'm sorry for what I said when I was hungry.

Workout: Alleviate Pain

Hold each stretch for 45 seconds and go through twice.
Equipment: mat

Child's pose to left and right
Cobra
Thread the needle, right
Thread the needle, left
Downward-facing dog
Wide legs, interlace hands behind, forward fold
Crescent moon, right
Crescent moon, left
Cross-body shoulder stretch, right
Cross-body shoulder stretch, left
Neck rotations

Triangle pose, right
Triangle pose, left
Humble warrior, right
Humble warrior, left
Bridge pose with arms under
Mountain pose to forward fold
Knee hugs on ground
Shoulder stand
Full-body stretch

Child's pose to left and right
Cobra
Thread the needle, right
Thread the needle, left
Downward-facing dog
Wide legs interlace hands behind forward fold
Crescent moon, right
Crescent moon, left
Cross-body shoulder stretch, right
Cross-body shoulder stretch, left
Neck rotations
Triangle pose, right
Triangle pose, left

Food

Breakfast: Sweet Potato Toast with Avocado and Egg (page 241)

Morning Snack

Lunch: California Veggie Bowl (page 262)

Afternoon Snack

Dinner: Teriyaki Tuna with Roasted Green Beans and Soba (page 273)

Evening Protein Snack

Daily Task

What can you do today to add value to someone else's life? It could be helping with groceries, giving them a call, bringing them flowers, or offering to help with something that you know will make a difference in their life. Don't feel that you are imposing on someone—we all love people reaching out and offering to give us a hand or show their affection.

Day 22

With all these nice acts of kindness and empowerment, you should be feeling all tingly inside. If not, you will be after this next workout, from the burn! Today we are targeting your upper body and those stubborn areas that are harder to tone.

> I don't want to look skinny. I want to look like I can kick your ass.

Workout: Targeted Upper Body

Stacked workouts: 1st and 2nd exercise; 1st, 2nd, and 3rd exercise; 1st, 2nd, 3rd, and 4th exercise; and so on. Rounds 1 and 2 are separate.

30 seconds of work / 10 seconds of rest
Equipment: mat, weights

Round 1
Across-body bicep curl to both arms front raise
High plank with alternating arm lift to side
Standing single rows to elbow pulls
Swinging leg drops
5-second hold narrow push-up to 5 narrow push-ups
V-sit crunches

Round 2
Arms out in front to elbows at 180 degrees
Expanding tabletops
Lying-down overhead tricep dips with leg drops
Palms face forward and pulses
Walk out to push-up
Shoulder taps

Food

Breakfast: Turkey and Kale Breakfast Bake (page 247)
Morning Snack
Lunch: Mango Shrimp Tacos (page 254)
Afternoon Snack
Dinner: Lemon Parmesan Salmon Zoodles (page 283)
Evening Protein Snack

Daily Task

Write out twenty affirmations. This may take you five minutes or, if you are being picky and hard on yourself, twenty-five minutes. Get Post-it notes or different pieces of paper and write a different affirmation on each one that is empowering and positive—something that's going to get you fired up in the morning. What you speak becomes your reality, so feed your mind with all the good words about you and your strengths.

DAYS 23–30

Shopping List

Dairy and Protein

Chicken breast, boneless and skinless (½ pound)

Eggs, large (½ dozen)

Fish: halibut (one 5-ounce fillet), tuna (two 4-ounce steaks)

Greek yogurt, unsweetened nonfat (if needed, 16-ounce container)

Mozzarella cheese, shredded (1 small bag, if needed)

Provolone cheese, deli sliced (⅛ pound)

Tofu, firm (one 16-ounce container)

Produce

Apples (3)

Arugula (1 container or bunch)

Avocado (1)

Baby spinach (one 5-ounce container)

Banana (1)

Bell pepper, red (1) and yellow (1)

Blueberries (one 4.4-ounce container)

Broccoli (1 head or 4 cups florets)

Button mushrooms (one 5-ounce container)

Cucumber (1)

Fingerling potatoes (6 ounces)

Grape tomatoes (1 container)

Herbs, fresh: basil (1 small container), cilantro (1 bunch), dill (1 small container), rosemary (1 small container, if needed), thyme (1 small container, if needed)

Oranges (2)

Peaches (2 small)

Shallot (1 small)

Zucchini (1)

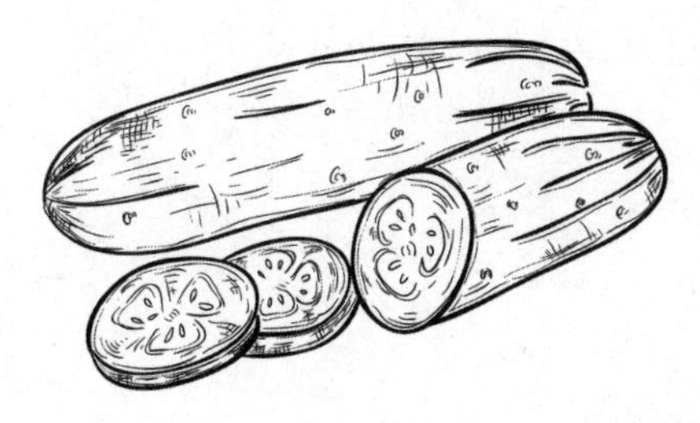

Meal Prep Plan

Day 23: Before you begin, prep hard-boiled eggs for snacks (if desired) and 1 cup dry brown rice. Prepare Blueberry Greek Yogurt Pancakes (1 portion in fridge/2 in freezer), and Greek Power Bowl with Shrimp (in fridge).

Day 27: Prepare Tofu Veggie Scramble and Sheet Pan Shrimp and Broccoli, and grill chicken for Grilled Chicken and Peach Salad (refrigerate all).

Fresh Prep: If possible, prepare these recipes right before you plan to enjoy them: Pesto Tuna Wraps (can be made the night before), Apple Pie Smoothie Bowl, Halibut and Veggie Skewers (make ½ the recipe), and Reboot Spinach and Almond Butter Smoothie.

Plan your snacks: Choose what appeals to you from the list on pages 140–141, planning for three per day.

Day 23

Get your mind focused today and give your soul positive words of affirmation: "I am going to slay today's workout. Yes!" We are strictly working on that butt today; although those glutes take a while to build, we are going to get started with that process. Level up and grab those weights!

> Diamonds were a girl's best friend
> until leggings happened.

Workout: Build That Butt

Stacked workouts: 1st and 2nd exercise; 1st, 2nd, and 3rd exercise; 1st, 2nd, 3rd, and 4th exercise; and so on. Rounds 1 and 2 are separate.

30 seconds of work / 15 seconds of rest
Equipment: mat, weights

Round 1
Reverse lunge to narrow deadlift
Diagonal donkey kicks, 15 seconds each leg
Leg hammer curl, 15 seconds each leg
Bridge pulses
Repeaters, 15 seconds each leg
In-and-out jumps with squat

Round 2
Standing leg across knee single squats, 15 seconds each leg
Wide deadlift
Tiptoe alternating reverse lunge
Squat pulses, arms in front
Standing leg pulses, 15 seconds each leg
Split lunges

Food

Breakfast: Apple Pie Smoothie Bowl (page 245)
Morning Snack
Lunch: California Veggie Bowl (page 262)
Afternoon Snack
Dinner: Teriyaki Tuna with Roasted Green Beans and Soba (page 273)
Evening Protein Snack

Daily Task

Call up an old friend. I am almost certain that you have a friend who hasn't heard from you in a while because it's "never the right time," thanks to delays and distractions. No more distractions today; the time is now. If it's late, send them a message to schedule a time to chat on the phone. If you don't, another day will pass, and remember, it's all about taking the first step right now. Reconnect, stay in contact, and make the effort to maintain relationships throughout your life. And if you are great at this already, reach out to someone with whom you might not be that close and build a stronger bond there.

Day 24

Today might be the day you invite your friends over or share this workout with them because, oh, are we going to feel the burn and be walking funny tomorrow! Yep, this inner and outer thigh workout is sure going to wake up all the muscles in your legs. I encourage you to add in resistance bands to get the most out of today's workout.

> Failure is not the opposite of success. It's part of it.

Workout: Inner and Outer Thigh Burn

45 seconds of work / 15 seconds of rest. Go through the whole sequence and then repeat from the beginning.
Equipment: mat, optional weights and resistance bands

Lying down, top leg over bottom leg, lift up bottom leg, right
Lying down, top leg over bottom leg, lift up bottom leg, left
Sumo squat, touch ground, then lift heels
Side lunge pulse, right
Side lunge pulse, left
Wide deadlifts
Front 45-degree leg swing, right
Front 45-degree leg swing, left
Bridge knee in-and-outs, twice
Squat to bent-leg lift, right

Squat to bent-leg lift, left
Side steps
Plie pulses

Food

Breakfast: Blueberry Greek Yogurt Pancakes (page 237)

Morning Snack

Lunch: Lemon Parmesan Salmon Zoodles (page 283)

Afternoon Snack

Dinner: Blueberry Balsamic Turkey Meatballs (page 266)

Evening Protein Snack

Daily Task

Make a vision board. It's time to get creative, make a mess, and glue stuff together! A vision board gets you focused on what you are striving toward and keeps you on track. It is a visual reminder each day of your purpose, the excitement to reach your goals, and your accountability to reach them. Find pictures in magazines or print them off the internet and use an actual poster board. There is a difference when you make something with your hands rather than just making something on a computer, so get your hands dirty. I suggest making one for yourself, and, if you are in a relationship, make one with your partner too so you can see their goals and check that you are both on the same page.

Day 25

You're closing in on the final days of the challenge, and I'm sure you're excited and also nervous about what's next. I have you covered, because this program just keeps on going! Every day I have a new workout for you, with new recipes every month, motivation, and a great community to keep you on track. Visit ICanFeelTheBurn.com for a free seven-day trial!

> Falling down is an accident; staying down is a choice.

Workout: Toned Abs and Calorie Cardio

Circuit workout: Do each round twice before moving to next round.

30 seconds of work / 15 seconds of rest
Equipment: mat

Round 1
Halfway sit-up pulses
Opposite mountain climbers
Plank in-and-out jumps
Leg drop circles

Round 2
Curtsy lunge with kick, right
Curtsy lunge with kick, left
Fast bicycles
Low plank to high plank

Round 3
Alternating elbow-to-knee oblique crunch
Dolphin plank leg lifts
V-sit overhead claps
High knees

Round 4
Russian twists double pulse
Straight-leg sit-up
Fast feet to tuck jump
Wide-leg forward fold, straight back to rise

Food

Breakfast: No-Bake Lime Coconut Protein Bites (page 249)

Morning Snack

Lunch: Greek Power Bowl with Shrimp (page 264)

Afternoon Snack

Dinner: Halibut and Veggie Skewers (page 281)

Evening Protein Snack

Daily Task

Choose a date to do something that is scary to you. You know what that thing is right in your gut, so say it out loud and declare you are going to make it happen no matter what fear you have, because the other side of fear is joy! Instead of procrastinating and making excuses as to why you can't start something, pick the date that you are going to start that thing you have been putting off. Now, this does not mean pick a date to think about what to start—decide this now and then commit to it, preferably in the next ninety days.

Day 26

If you aren't in the habit of checking out your muscles, this is your day! It's time to get the pump on with your biceps and triceps! Or, as we like to call that stubborn area under your arms, the bingo wings!

> Sometimes you win, and sometimes you learn.

Workout: Bicep, Shoulder, and Tricep Tone

Stacked workouts: 1st and 2nd exercise; 1st, 2nd, and 3rd exercise; 1st, 2nd, 3rd, and 4th exercise; and so on. Rounds 1 and 2 are separate.

30 seconds of work / 10 seconds of rest
Equipment: mat, weights

Round 1
Inchworms to narrow push-up
Bicep in-and-outs
Arms back 45-degree pulses
Bicep curl with a pulse
Overhead 45-degree press
Shoulder shrugs

Round 2
Overhead tricep extension
Arnold press
Alternating diagonal arm extensions
Single hammer curl to double hammer curl
Alternating high plank row to tricep extensions
Halfway body weight tricep dip hold

Food

Breakfast: Turkey and Kale Breakfast Bake (page 247)
Morning Snack
Lunch: Veggie Lover's Chili (page 260)
Afternoon Snack
Dinner: Blueberry Balsamic Turkey Meatballs (page 266)
Evening Protein Snack

Daily Task

It's time to journal! Get out your notebook and just start writing or drawing what you feel and what happened today. Getting your emotions onto paper can be a great way to relieve stress and unwind. Spend fifteen or twenty minutes doing this, really reflecting on the day you had. Where were you spending your time and energy? Was it in a positive way or could you have spent your time more wisely? This is such a great way to self-reflect and learn where we can grow!

Day 27

It's time to grab those heavier weights today and get that lower body working for us. We always want to be using a heavier weight for the lower part of our body than we do for our arms, chest, and back. The legs and glutes are bigger muscles and therefore can carry more weight. Always use a different set of weights for the upper and lower body.

> If at first you don't succeed,
> fix your ponytail and try again.

Workout: Tone Up Lower Body

45 seconds of work / 15 seconds of rest. Go through the whole sequence and then repeat from the beginning.
Equipment: mat, weights

Reverse lunge to single-leg deadlift, right
Reverse lunge to single-leg deadlift, left
Sumo squats
Side lunge with leg lift, right
Side lunge with leg lift, left
Squat jump to front of mat and turn around
Alternating diagonal squat
Romanian deadlift, right
Romanian deadlift, left

Wide squat to wide deadlift
Single-leg bridge with leg extension, right
Single-leg bridge with leg extension, left
Calf raises
Alternating open hip squat

Food

Breakfast: Tofu Veggie Scramble (page 243)
Morning Snack
Lunch: Turkey Egg Roll in a Bowl (page 252)
Afternoon Snack
Dinner: Sheet Pan Shrimp and Broccoli (page 272)
Evening Protein Snack

Daily Task

Be creative. When was the last time you did some arts and crafts? Our brain is often so focused on what we have to do next that we forget to be in the moment. Paint a picture, knit a scarf, do a puzzle, or compose a song! This could be something you did as a child and haven't done for years, or it could be something you have been wanting to try. Today is the day!

Day 28

It's that day when you get to stretch and give your muscles some much needed TLC! You will reduce the soreness of your muscles by dedicating time both after each workout and once a week to stretch your body. Plus, it feels good too!

> Don't wait for someone to bring you flowers. Plant your own garden.

Workout: Unwind for Sore Muscles

Hold each stretch for 40 seconds. Go through twice.

Equipment: mat

Standing forward fold, holding on to opposite elbows
Wide forward fold, moving to each side
Supine twist, right
Supine twist, left
Butterfly pose
Figure 4 stretch, right
Figure 4 stretch, left
Standing quad stretch, right
Standing quad stretch, left
Calf stretch, right
Calf stretch, left

Cross-legged hip stretch, right
Cross-legged hip stretch, left
Pedal out downward-facing dog

Food

Breakfast: Reboot Spinach and Almond Butter Smoothie (page 235)
Morning Snack
Lunch: Pesto Tuna Wrap (page 250)
Afternoon Snack
Dinner: Light Tofu Thai Curry (page 279)
Evening Protein Snack

Daily Task

It's time for *you*. You are going to love today's task because who doesn't love a little pampering and self-care? Book yourself a massage, get your nails done, or try a facial. It could be as simple as painting your nails at home or taking a nice soak in your tub. You don't have to spend a lot of money to treat yourself to the self-care you deserve. The important part is that you fill up your cup so you can be the best version of you for others.

Day 29

We're coming in hot for the last couple of days, so let's keep the momentum high and our squats nice and low! If you started at one weight at the beginning of this thirty days, let's give it a go upping that today to show yourself how much you have improved!

> My outfit is inspired by the fact that I woke up forty minutes late this morning.

Workout: Flatten Abs and Strengthen Lower Body

Stacked workouts: 1st and 2nd exercise; 1st, 2nd, and 3rd exercise; 1st, 2nd, 3rd, and 4th exercise; and so on. Rounds 1 and 2 are separate.

30 seconds of work / 10 seconds of rest
Equipment: mat, optional weights

Round 1
Alternating forward lunge with twist to the front knee
Alternating 3 steps back deadlift
Across-the-body mountain climbers
Single-leg drop with a pulse
Diagonal kick pulses, 15 seconds each side
Hold dolphin plank

Round 2
Curtsy lunge pulses, 15 seconds each side
Reverse lunge to forward kick, 15 seconds each side
Heel touches
Narrow squat to alternating oblique crunch
High plank to touch opposite foot
Frog jump with pulse

Food

Breakfast: Tofu Veggie Scramble (page 243)
Morning Snack
Lunch: Grilled Chicken and Peach Salad (page 256)
Afternoon Snack
Dinner: Sheet Pan Shrimp and Broccoli (page 272)
Evening Protein Snack

Daily Task

Go for a mile run. Yes, I know we have gotten your workout in today! When was the last time you went for a run outside? Listen to some music, a podcast like the *It Takes Grit* podcast, or just the sounds of your environment while you run at your own pace. I suggest timing yourself, just to see where you are at, and then going for a mile run again in another two weeks. Keep track of your fitness level by regularly doing this—it's a great indicator of your cardiovascular health.

Day 30

And just like that, we're here. You've made it through, and you should be so proud of yourself! Give yourself a nice pat on the back and tell yourself you did a great job! We are going to end our thirty days together by getting really sweaty in a HIIT (high-intensity interval training) workout, so buckle up and let's do this! You have come so far—now is the time to cement this into your lifestyle so you can be healthy and fit forever. Let's continue our journey together over on the BURN by Rebecca Louise program! By joining our community you know you are going to stay on track and keep on seeing results!

> Every time you eat or drink, you are either feeding disease or fighting it.

Workout: Turn It Up HIIT

Circuit workout: Do each round twice before moving to next round.

30 seconds of work / 15 seconds of rest
Equipment: mat

Round 1
Jogging
Inchworms to a push-up
Bicycles
Mountain climbers

Round 2
High knees
Plank jacks
Sit-up twists
High-to-low plank

Round 3
Frog jumps
Booty kickers
Side lunges, right
Side lunges, left

Round 4
Punch forward in a squat
Alternating side kick with squat jump
Side steps
Downward punches with fast feet

Round 5
Burpee
Forward punches with fast feet
Curtsy lunge with forward kick, right
Curtsy lunge with forward kick, left

Round 6
Star jumps
Marching on spot
Crabwalk to plank
Tuck jumps

Round 7
Plank forward and backward
Squats
Alternating reverse lunge to front kick
Grapevine

Round 8
Jogging
Inchworms to a push-up
Bicycles
Mountain climbers

Round 9
High knees
Plank jacks
Sit-up twists
High-to-low plank

Round 10
Frog jumps
Booty kickers
Side lunges, right
Side lunges, left

Food

Breakfast: Blueberry Greek Yogurt Pancakes (page 237)
Morning Snack
Lunch: Pesto Tuna Wrap (page 250)
Afternoon Snack
Dinner: Dinner out! You've earned it!
Evening Protein Snack

Daily Task

Meditate. The best way to seal your 30-Day Level Up Challenge is by taking at least ten minutes today in a peaceful, quiet place to simply meditate and give your mind some loving. With everything you have been through over this challenge, the ups and downs with the great days and the ones that tested you, it's important to recognize that you are still here, you did your best, and you didn't give up. Go to a place where you can be alone, sit down comfortably, and just allow your mind to find peace. Breathe slowly and enjoy receiving self-awareness. You've earned this moment! Well done.

10

Long-Term Success and Going the Extra Mile

Never Give Up

Just because you can see the page doesn't mean you're on it! Let's end together, on the same page, with the mindset to create all the success you want in the world. Whatever that might look like for you, we are not leaving until it's been embedded into your brain, without it falling out tomorrow!

Attaining success is not complicated, difficult, or challenging, because you already know what to do—follow the steps that have already been laid out and go the extra mile. Most people just aren't committed to "doing the do," so when you simply follow through, you will see how great it feels to pick up momentum in your journey. From losing extra pounds, to running a marathon, to building a side business . . . it's all there for you to take.

For me, quitting is not an option and has never been one. Maybe it's my pride, my ego, or (I like to think) just the sheer determination to make it work—whatever the reason, there is no plan B. I want to get you to that point, too. Here's how you're going to do it:

Know that you can't fail, as long as you don't give up.
Everything really is on you. It doesn't matter what other people think unless you allow their thinking to influence your actions. Sometimes when you wait for something for so long, you start to question if it will ever happen, so act quickly in taking the first step and keep trying. If you quit, it definitely won't ever happen!

I believe that anyone can do anything if they are given enough time and simply refuse to quit. That's the catch: Most people give up or don't do enough during the small amount of time they are on the planet to make it happen for them. It's inevitable that if you never give up, something good will come from your efforts.

Come back to your "why" when you feel like giving up.
How can you face yourself in the mirror knowing that you didn't achieve what you set out to because you quit? Not because you were not good enough, didn't know enough, or weren't capable, *just because you quit*! And if you have quit on something, right now, it's not too late, because you are still here! Start it up again and then you'll realize that you didn't quit after all; you just took a break.

Expect things to go really wrong.
Yes! This is just life testing you to see how much you want something. All you have to do is complete the task and pass the test, and you are on to the next chapter of your life and closer to where you want to be! The story you've created in your head is that everything is easy for everyone else apart from you, which is just your excuse for not

doing it. I don't know one successful person who has had an easy ride. Remember, you haven't come this far just to come this far.

Do it even when it's really hard.

This is just the universe testing you to see if you are ready for the next great things in your life. It's a reward for *leveling up*! Expect things to be super hard, be prepared for rejection, and be ready for the weight you can barely lift. Set yourself up for success by knowing that nothing that comes easy lasts. In moments of difficulty, push even harder, because you will need that extra push to get over the hump and onto the next stage of your journey. Don't quit in times of hardship; just level up, be more, and pass the universe's tests with flying colors!

So what if you mess up?

We all fuck up. My gosh, I have made so many mistakes and acted in a way that wasn't my best. What can we do with this—learn from it, get better, and move on, or live in a state of "what if," and "I can't believe I did that"? No, fuck that! You are human; we are not perfect. Give yourself grace, take it as something that needed to happen to shape who you are today, and use it to help you grow and flourish into the most amazing you there is!

Tips for Staying on Track

Fitness

Grab yourself a fitness buddy who will keep you accountable. A real friend will tell you when you're being lazy and get you off the couch and into your workout pants. This is the type of person you want: someone who wants to work out just as much as you do. I suggest finding someone with whom you are not overly familiar, maybe a new person from the gym or from my app community.

Find a class, workout, or exercise style that you love. If you dread going because you don't like it, then you are less likely to go. If you haven't found it yet, keep going and trying as many as it takes until you find the one that fits you. No excuses—you must pick something, so search for the one you enjoy the most.

Nutrition

Prepare your meals ahead of time and plan out what you are going to cook for the week. Prepping your meals and putting them in the freezer will be a game changer to keep you eating healthy.

Limit the takeout meals and dinners out, and when you do go out, remember to choose a rainbow-colored dinner. Make the effort to cook a nice meal at home, put the phones away, light a candle, and enjoy dinner. This will save you money and calories!

Stock up on healthy snacks that are ready and available to take with you. There are so many apps and services that will actually go and do your shopping for you. I use Instacart, which is an incredible app that delivers your groceries in two hours! This is a lifesaver for me—I have no excuses not to stock my cupboards with healthy foods.

Don't forget to plan your post-workout recovery shakes and supplements when setting out your meals. You are an athlete, and you should look after your body like one!

Motivation

The most crucial part to getting results is your mind. Changing the way you think brings about other changes—if you start to see things as positive, then you become positive. For this to happen you must immerse yourself in learning everything you can about leadership and personal development. Make it part of your daily routine. Keep reading twenty minutes of a personal development book every day. Make notes and absorb the information. Listen to podcasts that set your soul on fire and keep you believing and pushing for your goals. Check back in with your why, and make sure this still really is your why. (Hint: If you're not doing what you said you would be doing, then my guess is you haven't found your true why. Search again.) When the why is strong enough, the how is easy!

Connect with your goals to find your burning desire. What will it look like, feel like, and sound like to achieve those goals? Through the power of visualization, you can become emotionally connected to the outcome, which will drive you to get through the discomfort and make it happen. Daydream every day, see it, believe it, do the work, and don't give up when it gets hard. Your success is right around the corner.

Time Management

You must get organized! Create a daily schedule that includes all your non-negotiables: meal prep, workouts, self-care, personal development, and visualization. Without a schedule, life will take away your goals, so create your plan and stick to it no matter what.

Set daily goals that add up throughout the week to help you achieve your outcome and result. Remember, the goal is not to run a marathon—that is the outcome. The goal is to run two to three times a week to train so that you can complete the 26 miles. Each night, write your daily goals for the next day, then get up and smash them with no excuses as to why you couldn't. All excuses have the same value: zero.

If it helps to set alarms on your phone to remind you to eat, get a sweat on, or take time for yourself, then do that. I don't know how anyone goes through life without a diary! A daily log is essential for seeing where you are, what you need to do that day, and where your time is going.

How Are You Thinking? Breaking the Victim Mentality

There have been times when I have had a meltdown, yet I've turned to smile for the camera just to put my best face forward. I make the choice to be positive and change my mindset, so posting something negative on social media about how bad the traffic was or that my dinner at last night's restaurant was cold does not align with my values.

I see a lot of moaning, complaining, and victim mentality as I scroll social media, which really does not help you or your audience. Give up posting those attention-seeking "*Oh, it's just been one of those rough days*" statuses—it just makes your friends and family worry about you and it doesn't change anything! It is much better to share how you felt and what you did to overcome it. "Last week wasn't easy for me! I decided to take a couple of deep breaths, go for a brisk walk with a friend, try out a new restaurant, and after writing down all the things I was grateful for, I wasn't in as much pain." It's amazing what you can do when you start to think positively and how you can give back! Take action to find the solution and you can help others who are struggling with the same thing.

There is no shame in struggling with life—we all do. Find your solution, get better, and then share with the world so you add value. If you need help, send a direct message or talk to a friend or family member. You can be real while being positive and offering solutions. There is definitely no need to complain—you are too blessed to be stressed. You are alive!

Throughout the day you have X amount of energy, which we will visualize as balloons. Let's say you have seven (because that's my lucky number!). For instance, I wake up and Alphie has pissed on the bathroom mat for the third time this week. I get annoyed that the first thing I have to do is a chore, so I'm already boiled up. I head into the kitchen to make my morning smoothie and realize my boyfriend took my favorite flavor to work with him. Now I'm angry at both dog and boyfriend! Because I'm heated up, I forget to put the lid on the blender and smoothie mix ends up all over the ceiling, so I start crying and after thirty minutes of being awake I've burst three balloons, and I haven't even put my contact lenses in yet!

Now, let's look at it differently, which is going to save you thousands of "energy balloons" and is super simple to do. Alphie pisses in the bathroom—wow! What a clever boy, trying to use the bathroom, just like mummy! Ah, the boyfriend took my shake, so now I get to try a new flavor today. Smoothie all over the ceiling? This is going to make a great Instagram post! From annoyed, frustrated, and negative to calm, happy, and funny. When you look at things differently, the things you look at will change.

Limit "Venting" and Focus on the Solution

Do you have that friend who just saps your energy? Or worse, does your complaining do that to someone else? It's time to create boundaries, focus on solutions, and save your sanity!

If your friend is complaining about something or needs advice, ask them what they are looking for: Do they just want a listening ear and someone to rant at? Or are they looking for a solution and/or feedback to their complaint or problem? Wait until you know what they need and then go ahead and give them that. I think ranting is fine, just not if it's the same topic over and over, so after one or two of these conversations, it's time to shut it down. If someone asks for your help, does not implement it, and keeps coming back to talk, feel free to say that you've listened and offered solutions, and if they don't want to take action to solve the problem or listen to your advice, you don't want to hear it again. Not only will this create a boundary for you and save your energy, it will also help the other person take action; otherwise you will end up enabling them to repeat their behavior.

And this works great the other way around, too. It's okay to sometimes say "Hey, I'm just looking to rant and rave for twenty minutes; can you just humor me and listen?" Or you can ask a friend for advice and a solution for the challenges you are facing right now, then go ahead and do it. Don't be that person who always complains and never makes anything better. Vent, ask for advice, then act to make the changes you need!

How great would this world be if you could take the things you've learned in this book and share them with friends? "I just wanted to let you know that this is what I have been going through and this is my solution to overcome my challenge. What do you think? I am going to implement it. I wanted to let you know and ask for your support." There you go: All parties' time is saved, the focus is positive change, and no one is sucking the energy out of one another. Hooray!

Accept Feedback

Take the feedback you are given. There is no need to cross your arms and frown; we are not toddlers anymore. Your inner critic wants to get defensive and put your guard up when it comes to hearing what you perceive as negative thoughts and comments. Get obsessed and addicted to feedback and criticism because it will allow you to elevate to a whole new level.

Anyone who doesn't want to listen to critical feedback will get stuck. It doesn't matter if you agree or not; it's always worth listening because you will get something from it if you choose to. Use this free knowledge to get better.

Now, if you are not ready that day to listen to feedback, that's okay, and you can set boundaries to say you are not willing to receive. However, in a new day and different mindset, return to that possibly difficult feedback. That grit you have discovered is not going to let you quit on your dreams and success just because of someone else's opinion, so put that grit you have created to the test and hear it all. Not listening to feedback will stunt your growth. You don't have to agree, so let your ego go and open your ears to listen to what could be holding you back from your next chapter.

Live with Gratitude

Wherever you are in life, have gratitude for the space you are in right at this moment. Have gratitude that you picked up this book, read it, and now have new information stored in your mind that can help you own your life.

When it feels like life is getting to be too much, return to what makes you grateful. List in your head or write down all the things for which you are thankful. You can always find at least three things that make you appreciate life and what you have. It could be that you are breathing, that you have your family, or that you ate something yummy that day. There is no need to play the victim and not list anything. We all have things we can appreciate in life and when we look for them, acknowledge them, and breathe into it, the light starts to appear and the tension in our shoulders eases away. We are too blessed to be stressed, and when we choose to be grateful and positive, our life seems a little easier to manage. That grit appears every time to keep us on track.

At the end of the day, you have two choices when these things happen to you: You can hide away in a shell and think "Why me?" or you can get in the mindset to learn from this experience and move forward.

Choosing your desired result should be easy. In Chapter 1, I asked you to write down your biggest goals. Have you taken at least one step to get closer to the goals yet? And if not, when are you going to take that step? In my world there are no excuses, so it's just a matter of when, not if, you will take that step and start achieving the life you want.

Now you have the skills, the vision, and the plan. It's time to take action! All you need to do is take the first step and keep going!

Use the tools in this book with no excuses and know that the choice is yours to make it happen for yourself. Go make yourself proud and *level up to a new standard!*

Tasks

- Reflect back on this book and list three things you have learned about controlling your mind and thoughts that have set you free. Now go back and read those sections through with a more teachable attitude.

- Write out how you are going to behave and react to experiences in the future that might once have upset you. Example: "The next time I hear negativity from someone I am not going to allow their energy to affect who I am and what I do because I have complete control of my thoughts and actions."

- *Celebrate!* Get off your butt right now—yes, this will not be ingrained in you without you moving your body and feeling it with every cell. Jump up and down, shout "Yes!," dance, and smile. Now let's get to work on crushing your goals; all you need is within you!

11

The Recipes

Breakfast Recipes

Reboot Spinach and Almond Butter Smoothie

Start your day with a balanced green smoothie with just the right amount of protein, plus a little sweetness to curb those sugar cravings! Packed full of antioxidants, this fast, easy, no-mess breakfast will reboot your energy levels and boost your immune system.

1 medium banana
½ cup baby spinach
2 tablespoons vanilla protein powder
1 tablespoon almond butter
1 cup coconut water

1. Combine the banana, spinach, protein powder, and almond butter in a blender with the coconut water and a few ice cubes. Blend until desired consistency is reached. I like mine thicker, so I add one or two extra ice cubes!
2. Pour into a tall glass and enjoy!

Prep time: 5 minutes
Makes: 1 (16-ounce) serving
Serving size: 1 smoothie

Smoked Salmon Avocado Toast

This "knife and fork" sandwich is a super-quick, satisfying meal that makes breakfast feel like a special occasion. Enjoy it as is or have fun with the toppings—try thin slices of your favorite raw veggies, roasted bell peppers, capers, or feta cheese to mix it up.

1 slice 100% whole wheat bread
½ avocado
1 tablespoon fresh lemon juice
1 teaspoon hemp seeds
1- to 2-oz piece smoked salmon
1 large hard-boiled egg, sliced
½ cup arugula
½ cup halved grape tomatoes
1 tablespoon sliced scallions
Salt and freshly ground pepper

1. Toast the bread to your liking.
2. In a small bowl, mash the avocado, lemon juice, and hemp seeds. Season with salt and pepper to taste.
3. Spread the avocado mash on the toast, then top with smoked salmon, sliced egg, arugula, tomatoes, and scallions. Cheers!

Shortcut: Prep the avocado mash the night before and store in an airtight container with plastic wrap pressed tightly to the surface of the avocado mixture to prevent browning. Or skip the mashing step and just pile everything onto the toast, and enjoy.

Prep time: 10 minutes
Makes: 1 sandwich | Serving size: 1 sandwich

Blueberry Greek Yogurt Pancakes

Who can resist a plate of fluffy, sweet pancakes, especially when they're packed with healthy protein and ready to go when you are? Make this ultimate meal prep recipe ahead and freeze individual portions for your on-the-go lifestyle, or mix up a double batch for the family on Sunday morning!

1 cup whole-wheat pastry flour
¼ cup vanilla protein powder
1 tablespoon baking powder
1 teaspoon cane sugar
Pinch of salt
1 cup almond milk
2 large eggs
1 teaspoon vanilla extract
½ cup unsweetened nonfat Greek yogurt
¼ cup fresh blueberries
1 teaspoon coconut oil, for the pan

For each serving:

1 teaspoon butter
1 teaspoon honey
1 teaspoon sliced almonds

1. In a large bowl, whisk the whole-wheat pastry flour, protein powder, baking powder, cane sugar, and salt until combined. Set aside.
2. In a small bowl, whisk the almond milk, eggs, and vanilla extract. Add this mixture to the dry ingredients and mix well. Gently fold in the Greek yogurt and blueberries.
3. Heat a griddle or 12-inch skillet over medium heat and coat with coconut oil. Spoon ¼ cup of batter onto the pan for each pancake and cook until bubbles start to form around the edges. Flip and cook until golden brown. Repeat with remaining batter.

4. Serve three pancakes topped with 1 teaspoon each of butter, honey, and sliced almonds.

Note: To store your pancakes, let them cool completely, then wrap individual servings of three pancakes in plastic wrap and store in the freezer. To reheat, unwrap pancakes, place them on a microwave-safe plate, cover with a paper towel, and microwave at full power for 1 or 2 minutes, or until hot.

Prep time: 5 minutes | Cook time: 15 minutes
Makes: 9–10 pancakes | Serving size: 3 pancakes

Parmesan Veggie Frittata

Spinach is full of vitamin K, vitamin B2, and vitamin C, all of which are great for skin, hair, and bone growth. Broccoli and eggs bring protein power, with mushrooms and onions joining the party for fiber and flavor. Topped with a sprinkle of melty Parmesan, this calcium- and vitamin-rich, meal-prep-ready frittata will soon be your favorite way to start the day!

1 teaspoon extra-virgin olive oil
½ cup broccoli florets, roughly chopped
½ cup sliced button mushrooms
¼ cup diced yellow onion
1 clove garlic, minced
2 cups baby spinach
5 large eggs, beaten
2 tablespoons shredded Parmesan
Salt and freshly ground pepper

For serving:
1 slice whole wheat toast (per serving)
1 cup mixed berries

1. Preheat oven to broil.
2. Heat the olive oil in a small oven-safe skillet over medium heat. Sauté the broccoli, mushrooms, onions, and garlic until the onions and mushrooms begin to brown, stirring frequently, for about 3 minutes. Season with a pinch of salt and pepper, add the spinach, and cover with a lid for 1 minute to steam the spinach. Remove the lid and stir for 1 minute more.
3. Pour the beaten eggs over the veggie mixture, reduce the heat to medium-low, and

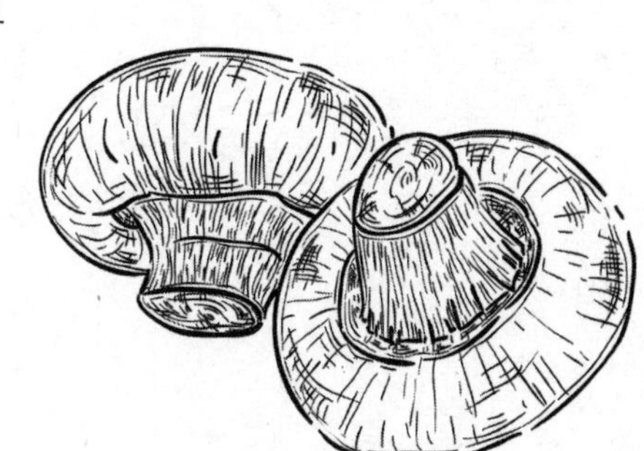

cook for about 4 minutes, or until the eggs are set around the edges. Top with Parmesan.

4. Transfer the skillet to the oven and broil for 2 or 3 minutes, or until the eggs are puffed, golden brown, and set in the middle. Transfer to a cutting board, slice in half, and enjoy with toast and berries.

Shortcut: Save time by using chopped frozen broccoli in this recipe.

Note: This frittata is great hot, warm, or cold. Cool completely before storing in the fridge for up to 5 days. To freeze individual portions, cool completely, then wrap tightly in plastic wrap. Heat refrigerated or frozen frittata in the microwave in 1-minute increments until hot.

Prep time: 10 minutes | Cook time: 10 minutes
Makes: 1 frittata | Serving size: ½ of frittata

Sweet Potato Toast with Avocado and Egg

Level up your meal prep game with this delicious breakfast! Sweet potato toast is the perfect bread alternative when you're looking to mix it up, and you'll have a few extra slices for snacks, too. Topped with a creamy avocado mash featuring a sneaky serving of extra veggies, plus eggs for protein and staying power, it's irresistible!

For the sweet potato toasts:
1 large, tubular sweet potato

For the avocado mash:
½ cup frozen peas, defrosted
½ avocado
¼ cup unsweetened nonfat Greek yogurt
1 tablespoon fresh lemon juice
1 scallion, thinly sliced
½ teaspoon chili powder
Salt and freshly ground pepper

For each serving:
2 hard-boiled eggs, sliced
Hot sauce, to taste
1 cup fresh fruit

1. Preheat oven to 375°F. Line a large baking sheet with parchment paper.
2. Scrub the sweet potato and pat it dry. Cut a small piece off each end, then stand it up on your cutting board and carefully cut ¼-inch lengthwise slices (or use a mandoline).
3. Bake the sweet potato slices on the parchment-lined baking sheet for 20 minutes, turning once, until they are just tender.
4. Meanwhile, in a small bowl, mash the peas, avocado, yogurt, lemon juice, and scallion. Stir in the chili powder, then season to taste with salt and pepper.
5. When you're ready to serve, pop 2 slices of sweet potato toast into your toaster and toast just until heated through and lightly browned. Top each slice with 2 tablespoons of avocado mash and

a sliced hard-boiled egg. Drizzle with hot sauce, and enjoy with a side of fresh fruit. Yum!

Note: This recipe yields enough sweet potato toast for 2 breakfasts plus a couple of snacks. Be sure to cool the toasts completely before storing in an airtight container in the fridge. At snack time, enjoy one toast topped with almond butter and fruit, avocado and smoked salmon, or hummus and sliced bell peppers. The possibilities are endless! You'll have enough avocado mash for 2 breakfasts. Store leftovers in an airtight container in the fridge with a layer of plastic wrap pressed to the surface to keep it from browning. Double the avocado mash recipe and you'll have enough dip for even more snacks—it's delicious with fresh veggie dippers or seed crackers.

Prep time: 10 minutes
Cook time: 20 minutes
Makes: 7 sweet potato toasts; ½ cup avocado mash
Serving size: 2 sweet potato toasts plus ¼ cup avocado mash

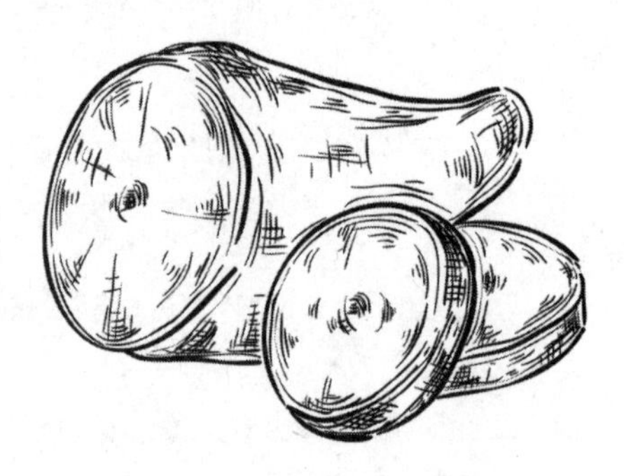

Tofu Veggie Scramble

This satisfying morning scramble will check all your boxes when it comes to flavor and protein. Fuel your body with loads of vitamins and nutrients to conquer your day and save time when doing the dishes—this one cooks up in one pan!

½ block firm tofu (8 ounces)
2 teaspoons extra-virgin olive oil
1 garlic clove, minced
1½ cups diced white button mushrooms (about 3½ ounces)
½ cup diced red onion
½ cup diced red bell pepper
1 teaspoon soy sauce
Salt and freshly ground pepper

For each serving:
½ cup chopped grape tomatoes
¼ avocado, sliced
1 slice 100% whole wheat toast
1 orange, sliced

1. Drain the tofu and squeeze it dry, then crumble it into pieces. I like to make mine in bigger pieces as it leaves the tofu a bit softer in the middle while cooking.
2. Heat the olive oil in a large nonstick skillet over medium-high heat. Add the garlic and cook for 30 seconds, then add the mushrooms, onion, and bell pepper. Sauté for 2 minutes, then add the crumbled tofu and soy sauce and cook for 5 minutes more, stirring frequently. Season with salt and pepper.
3. Serve half of the scramble immediately, topped with

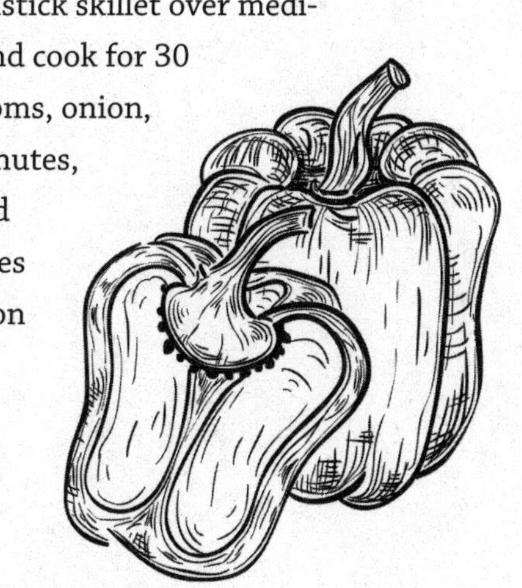

tomatoes and sliced avocado, with whole wheat toast and orange slices on the side.

4. Store the other half of the scramble in an airtight container in the fridge for up to 3 days. Reheat in the microwave for 2 minutes before serving.

Note: Feeling spicy? This makes a great filling for breakfast tacos! Stir ½ teaspoon chili powder and a pinch of crushed red pepper flakes into the scramble when you add the tofu. Replace the toast with two small whole wheat tortillas, then pile on the tomato and avocado, drizzle with hot sauce, and enjoy!

Prep time: 10 minutes | Cook time: 10 minutes
Makes: 2 servings | Serving size: ½ of scramble

Apple Pie Smoothie Bowl

This refreshing smoothie bowl has all the amazing flavors of Thanksgiving! Try it when you want a sweet start plus lots of energy to take on your day!

½ cup unsweetened nonfat Greek yogurt
1 unpeeled apple, sliced into wedges
½ cup rolled oats
¼ cup baby spinach
1 tablespoon vanilla protein powder
1 teaspoon brown sugar
¼ teaspoon cinnamon

For serving:
1 tablespoon granola
1 tablespoon dried cranberries
1 teaspoon chia seeds

1. Combine the yogurt, apple, oats, spinach, protein powder, brown sugar, and cinnamon in a blender with a handful of ice cubes (if desired). Blend on low until combined, scraping the blender bowl down once or twice; then turn to high and blend until smooth.
2. Pour into a bowl, sprinkle with the granola, cranberries, and chia seeds, and enjoy immediately.

Kitchen Tip: Smoothies are so versatile! Modify the recipe depending on what you have in your fridge. Try swapping the apples with some tasty in-season berries, or switch up the toppings with different nuts, dried fruit, or hemp seeds.

Prep time: 5 minutes
Makes: 1 smoothie bowl
Serving size: 1 bowl

Berry Breakfast Pops

Satisfying your sweet tooth has never been easier! You can make these in no time and stay on track. Who said you can't have dessert for breakfast? These also make a great snack if you find yourself in front of the fridge at 1 AM.

1 cup unsweetened nonfat Greek yogurt
¼ cup vanilla protein powder
½ banana
½ cup chopped strawberries
½ cup blueberries
1 kiwi, peeled and chopped
1 cup granola
1 tablespoon honey

1. In a blender, combine the yogurt, protein powder, banana, strawberries, blueberries, and kiwi. Blend until smooth.
2. Divide the mixture evenly among four jumbo ice pop molds, leaving at least ½ inch of space at the top of each mold. Freeze, uncovered, for 10 minutes to firm up slightly.
3. Stir the granola and honey together in a small bowl, then spoon ¼ of the mixture into each mold.
4. Tap the mold gently on the countertop to settle the ingredients, then insert the sticks/covers and freeze for at least 12 hours.
5. To serve, run ice pop mold under warm water for a minute, then pull gently to release.

Note: You'll need a jumbo ice pop mold that holds at least ½ cup of liquid per mold to make this as a breakfast recipe. If your mold is smaller, make 6 to 8 popsicles and enjoy them as a refreshing snack.

Prep time: 15 minutes
Makes: 4 pops | Serving size: 1 pop

Turkey and Kale Breakfast Bake

I suggest cooking with turkey meat over beef—it has the same hearty, meaty taste with half the fat! This breakfast bake is easy to prepare, and it makes enough to freeze or share.

1 tablespoon coconut oil, divided, plus more for greasing pan
12 ounces 99% lean ground turkey
1 teaspoon dried thyme
½ teaspoon chili powder
1 clove garlic, minced
1 medium red onion, diced
1 large sweet potato, coarsely grated (about 3 cups)
2 cups chopped kale (about ½ bunch)
1 Granny Smith apple, peeled and finely chopped
1 cup cooked black beans, rinsed and drained
½ cup sliced scallions
8 large eggs
½ cup unsweetened almond milk
Salt and freshly ground pepper

pepper Optional, for serving:
Hot sauce
Sliced avocado

1. Preheat oven to 375°F. Grease a 9-inch square baking dish with coconut oil or cooking spray.
2. Heat 1½ teaspoons of the coconut oil in a large nonstick skillet over medium heat, then add the turkey, thyme, and chili powder. Season with salt and pepper and cook for about 5 minutes, stirring frequently, until the turkey is no longer pink; then drain and set aside in a bowl.
3. Add the remaining 1½ teaspoons of coconut oil to the same pan, and sauté the garlic, red onion, sweet potato, kale, and apple for about 5 minutes. Stir in the turkey, black beans, and scallions and remove from heat.

4. In a medium bowl, whisk the eggs and almond milk until well combined, then pour into the greased baking pan. Evenly spoon the turkey mixture into the eggs, and bake for 30 minutes, or until eggs are fully set.
5. Cool for 5 minutes, then slice into six pieces. Serve garnished with optional hot sauce and avocado, if desired. Store cooled leftovers in an airtight container in the refrigerator for up to 5 days, or wrap individual portions in plastic wrap and store in the freezer for up to 3 months. To reheat, place on a microwave-safe dish and heat on high power for 3 minutes, or until hot.

Shortcut: It's so easy to make this dish with pre-prepped veggies from your supermarket's produce department. Look for sweet potato "zoodles" to use instead of shredded sweet potato and purchase bagged, pre-washed chopped kale to cut your prep time to almost no time at all!

Prep time: 10 minutes
Cook time: 30 minutes
Makes: 1 (9-inch square) casserole
Serving size: 1/6 of casserole

No-Bake Lime Coconut Protein Bites

These bites are the perfect combination of protein, carbs, and healthy fats to keep you full of energy, and they pack and travel well, too. Keep them in the fridge so you can grab a couple for a quick breakfast on the run, or enjoy one for an afternoon pick-me-up!

1 cup raw cashews
1 cup packed pitted Medjool dates
½ cup vanilla protein powder
½ cup dried unsweetened coconut
2 teaspoons lime zest
2 tablespoons fresh lime juice

1. Pulse the cashews in a food processor or blender until they resemble coarse sand.
2. Add the dates and protein powder and process until a soft dough forms.
3. Add the coconut, lime zest, and lime juice and continue to process until well mixed.
4. Roll into 10 equal-size balls, about 1¾ inches each. Refrigerate until chilled. Store in the fridge for up to 1 week, or in the freezer for up to 3 months.

Prep time: 15 minutes
Makes: 10 bites | Serving size: 2 bites

Lunch Recipes

Pesto Tuna Wraps

This wrap is one of my favorites because I eat fish almost every day. Since I became pescatarian, it's my go-to protein. This wrap is *amazing* because it adds so much extra flavor.

For the tuna filling:

½ cup cooked navy (or cannellini) beans, rinsed and drained
1 tablespoon fresh lemon juice
2 teaspoons extra-virgin olive oil
1 (5-ounce) can solid white tuna, drained
Salt and freshly ground pepper

For the sandwiches:

2 whole wheat lavash wraps
2 slices provolone cheese
1 cup baby spinach, divided
½ cup chopped grape tomatoes, divided
¼ cup fresh basil leaves, divided

For serving:

2 oranges, sliced

1. Mash the beans, lemon juice, and olive oil with a fork in a medium bowl until smooth. Stir in the tuna and mix until well combined. Season to taste with salt and pepper.
2. Lay 1 lavash wrap on a cutting board and spread half of the tuna mixture over the center of the wrap. Top with 1 slice of provolone, followed by half of the spinach, tomatoes, and basil. Roll into a cylinder and serve with orange slices on the side. Store the remaining ingredients separately in airtight containers in the fridge.

Shortcut: For meal prep, make this recipe through step 1, and store the pre-measured ingredients in airtight containers for up to 3 days. When you're ready to make your lunch, continue with step 2 and enjoy! If you're packing a lunch to go, you can make this the night before and wrap it tightly in plastic wrap or foil.

Tip: For a vegan or vegetarian option, use 1½ cups of mashed chickpeas instead of white beans and tuna.

Prep time: 10 minutes
Makes: 2 servings | Serving size: 1 wrap

Turkey Egg Roll in a Bowl

Not all comfort food has to be bad for you! A deep-fried takeout favorite becomes a healthy, fiber-packed recipe that's perfect for meal prep, and bagged shredded cabbage and broccoli slaw mean less chopping and prep time for you. To spice things up, try a drizzle of sriracha or Chinese hot mustard.

1 tablespoon olive oil
½ pound 99% lean ground turkey
1 teaspoon toasted sesame oil
1 yellow onion, finely diced
2 cloves garlic, crushed
1 tablespoon finely chopped fresh ginger
1 (12-ounce) package broccoli slaw
2 cups shredded cabbage (about ½ package of coleslaw mix)
2 tablespoons reduced-sodium soy sauce, plus more to taste
2 teaspoons apple cider vinegar
1 cup mung bean sprouts
3 scallions, sliced, white and green parts separated
Salt and freshly ground pepper
2 cups cooked brown rice

1. Heat a large skillet over medium heat. Coat the pan with the olive oil, then add the turkey and cook until it's just beginning to brown, breaking it up with a spatula as you stir. Transfer the turkey to a bowl and set aside.
2. Add the sesame oil to the same skillet over medium-high heat. Sauté the onion for 5 minutes, then add the garlic and ginger and cook for 1 minute more. Stir in the broccoli slaw and shredded cabbage and cook for another minute.
3. Return the turkey to the skillet and stir in the soy sauce and vinegar. Add ¼ cup water, then stir and cover. Reduce the heat to low and cook for about 10 minutes, or until the broccoli slaw and

cabbage are cooked to desired tenderness. Stir in the bean sprouts and white parts of sliced scallions and cook for 1 minute more. Remove from heat and season to taste with salt, pepper, and a little more soy sauce if desired.

4. To assemble, divide the rice into three bowls and/or storage containers, then top each with an equal amount of the veggie/turkey mixture. Garnish with the sliced scallion greens.
5. Store leftovers in the refrigerator in airtight containers for up to 4 days or freeze individual portions for up to 3 months. (See page 289 for freezing tips.)

Shortcut: If you want to cut your prep time even more, look for frozen cubes of fresh garlic and ginger in the freezer department of your supermarket.

Prep time: 10 minutes
Cook time: 30 minutes
Makes: 3 bowls | Serving size: 1 bowl

Mango Shrimp Tacos

Spice up your afternoon with these zesty tacos! The fresh mango–black bean salsa adds a fruity zip to the flavorful, marinated shrimp.

For the shrimp:

1 tablespoon extra-virgin olive oil, divided
¼ cup cilantro, divided
1 teaspoon lime zest
Juice of one lime, divided
1 clove garlic, minced
¼ teaspoon cumin
10 ounces medium shrimp, peeled and deveined, thawed if frozen (about 20 shrimp)
Salt and freshly ground pepper

For the salsa:

½ cup diced mango
½ cup black beans
¼ cup diced red onion
¼ cup crumbled feta cheese
¼ cup grape tomatoes, quartered

For serving:

4 small whole wheat tortillas

1. Whisk 1 teaspoon of the olive oil, half of the cilantro, the lime zest, half of the lime juice, garlic, and cumin in a large bowl. Season with a pinch of salt and a little pepper, then stir in the shrimp. Cover and refrigerate while you make the salsa.
2. In a small bowl, combine the mango, black beans, red onion, feta, and tomatoes. Stir in the remaining cilantro; then add lime juice, salt, and pepper to taste.
3. Heat the remaining 2 teaspoons of olive oil in a large sauté pan over medium heat. Sauté the shrimp until opaque and pink, about 5 minutes.
4. To assemble the tacos, place about 6 shrimp in each tortilla and top with salsa. Serve immediately.

5. Store leftover shrimp and salsa in separate containers in the refrigerator for up to 3 days. To reheat, place shrimp and tortilla on a microwave-safe dish and heat for 45 seconds to 1 minute. Top with chilled mango salsa.

Shortcut: Frozen shrimp that's already peeled and deveined is a huge time-saver! Check the ingredients list to be sure the only ingredients are shrimp and salt—you don't want to add nasty preservatives to the menu! If you're really pressed for time, shop your supermarket's produce department for freshly prepared veggie or fruit salsa.

Kitchen Tip: Try making this recipe with a boneless, skinless chicken breast instead. Slice the chicken into thin strips, marinate, and sauté until cooked through.

Prep time: 5 minutes
Cook time: 20 minutes
Makes: 4 tacos
Serving size: 2 tacos

Grilled Chicken and Peach Salad

If you think salad can't be a filling, satisfying lunch, think again! This salad satisfies with a healthy dose of veggies, antioxidant-packed peaches, and flavorful grilled chicken. Grill the chicken while you slice the veggies and make the dressing, and this meal-prep friendly dish is ready in 20 minutes.

For the salad:

1 boneless, skinless chicken breast
1 teaspoon olive oil
2 cups arugula
1 cup grape tomatoes, halved
1 cup fresh peaches, sliced (about 2 small peaches)
2 tablespoons crumbled feta cheese
Salt and freshly ground pepper

For the dressing:

2 teaspoons extra-virgin olive oil
1 teaspoon apple cider vinegar
1 teaspoon Dijon mustard
1 teaspoon honey

1. Heat a grill or grill pan over medium-high heat and coat with cooking spray. Coat the chicken with the olive oil and season with a pinch of salt and pepper. Grill until the internal temperature reaches 165°F, about 10 minutes per side. Set aside to cool while you prepare the salad.
2. Combine the arugula, tomatoes, peaches, and feta in a large bowl. To make the dressing, whisk together the olive oil, vinegar, mustard, and honey in a small bowl. Add the dressing to the salad and toss to coat evenly.
3. Dice the chicken, add half of it to the salad, and enjoy!

Note: This recipe makes twice as much chicken as you need, so be mindful of those palm-size portions of protein! Pack up the extra chicken for a quick salad on the go or enjoy 2 ounces of chicken with a piece of fresh fruit as a healthy snack.

Kitchen Tip: Packing this salad up for meal prep? Put the dressing in the bottom of the container, then add the tomatoes, peaches, and chicken. Top with arugula and feta and store in the fridge for up to 2 days. When you're ready to eat, just shake and enjoy!

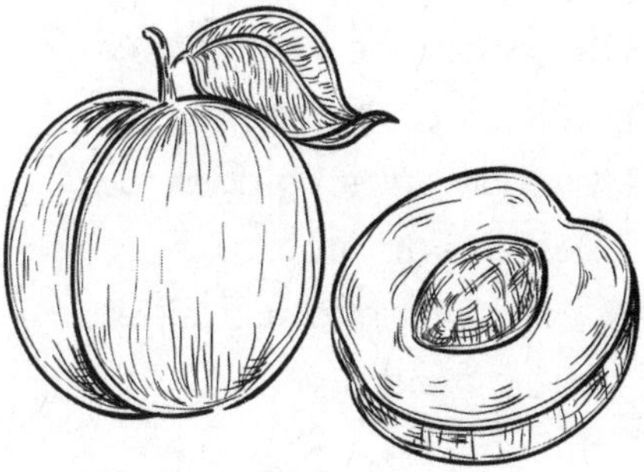

Prep time: 10 minutes
Cook time: 20 minutes
Makes: 1 salad/2 servings of chicken
Serving size: 1 salad/half of chicken

Sweet Tofu and Cauliflower Salad

This salad is perfect for a busy schedule. Tofu is a great substitute for meat because it contains a ton of vitamins and amino acids. It's great to have a salad in your repertoire that travels well and can be eaten cold. Enjoy this one anywhere!

For the tofu:

1 tablespoon soy sauce
1 tablespoon sesame oil
1 teaspoon rice wine vinegar
1 tablespoon honey
1 teaspoon fresh ginger root, peeled and grated
½ pound firm tofu, drained and patted dry

For the salad:

2 cups peeled and cubed butternut squash (1-inch cubes)
1 tablespoon olive oil
1 medium cauliflower head, cut into small florets
1 cup canned chickpeas, rinsed and drained
¼ cup chopped red onion
2 tablespoons prepared Asian ginger vinaigrette
½ cup red seedless grapes, halved
2 tablespoons thinly sliced scallions
Salt and freshly ground pepper

1. Preheat oven to 400°F. Whisk the soy sauce, sesame oil, rice wine vinegar, honey, and ginger in a medium bowl. Dice the tofu into 1-inch cubes and gently combine with the marinade. Set aside to marinate for about 10–15 minutes at room temperature while you prepare the veggies for the salad.
2. On a large, rimmed baking sheet lined with parchment paper, toss the squash cubes with the olive oil, then season lightly with salt and pepper to taste. Spread the marinated tofu cubes on another lined baking sheet. Place both in the oven and bake for 20 minutes, or until the squash is tender and the tofu is lightly browned. Set aside to cool slightly.

3. While the squash and tofu are roasting, set a steamer basket in a large pot with 2 cups of water and bring to a boil. Add the cauliflower, cover, and steam for 8 minutes, or until tender. Set aside to cool for 10 minutes.
4. Combine the steamed cauliflower, roasted squash, tofu, chickpeas, and red onions.
5. Add vinaigrette and mix until well combined. Stir in the grapes and scallions.
6. Divide salad between two large storage containers, and store in the refrigerator for up to 5 days.

Prep time: 15 minutes | Cook time: 35 minutes
Makes: 2 servings | Serving size: ½ of salad

Veggie Lover's Chili

Toss the ingredients for this easy, delicious chili in your slow cooker when you start your meal prep—it's an easy way to get a couple of meals going while you prep the rest. Store it in the freezer in individual portions and you'll never have to stray from your meal plan. What you eat is going to determine 80 percent of your results, and this chili is 100 percent going to give you a kickstart!

3 cups reduced-sodium vegetable broth
2 (15-ounce) cans black beans, rinsed and drained
2 (15-ounce) cans pinto beans, rinsed and drained
1 (14.5-ounce) can diced tomatoes
1 cup chopped onion
1 red bell pepper, seeded and chopped
2 cloves garlic, minced
2 tablespoons chili powder
1 tablespoon extra-virgin olive oil
1 teaspoon dried oregano
1 teaspoon ground cumin
1 teaspoon hot sauce, plus more to taste
1 cup cooked quinoa
Salt and freshly ground pepper

For each serving:

½ cup unsweetened nonfat Greek yogurt
1 teaspoon hemp seeds
Chopped cilantro, to taste
Lime wedge

1. In a slow cooker, combine the vegetable broth, black beans, pinto beans, tomatoes, onions, pepper, garlic, chili powder, olive oil, oregano, cumin, and hot sauce. Season with a pinch of salt and pepper. Stir to combine well, then cover and cook on high for 3 to 4 hours (or, if you're headed out for the day, cook on low for 6 to 8 hours).
2. Just before serving, stir the quinoa into the chili. Season to taste with salt, pepper, and a little more hot sauce, if desired.

3. Divide the chili evenly among 5 bowls and/or storage containers. When you're ready to serve, top with Greek yogurt, hemp seeds, cilantro, and a lime wedge.
4. Store leftovers in the fridge for up to 5 days, or in airtight containers in the freezer for up to 3 months.

Kitchen Tip: Want to spice up your life? Add more of your favorite hot sauce or red pepper flakes to each serving to get more of a kick, or add a seeded, diced jalapeno to the slow cooker with the rest of the ingredients.

Prep time: 10 minutes
Cook time: 3 to 4 hours (high) or 6 to 8 hours (low)
Makes: 5 servings | Serving size: 1/5 of recipe

California Veggie Bowl

This bowl is going to fuel your body with the vitamins and nutrients for energy to carry you through a busy day. The vegetables in this recipe are in season all year long, so it's easy to locate them at a local farmers' market or your favorite grocery store.

1 small sweet potato, peeled and cubed
1 teaspoon extra-virgin olive oil
4 cups arugula
½ cup cooked quinoa
1 cup canned black beans, rinsed and drained
1 cup grape tomatoes, halved
1 cup shredded carrots
1 avocado, sliced
2 tablespoons hemp seeds
1 lemon, halved
Salt and freshly ground pepper

1. Preheat oven to 425°F. Line a large, rimmed baking sheet with parchment paper.
2. Toss the sweet potato with the olive oil, and season with a pinch of salt and pepper. Spread in an even layer and bake for 15 minutes, or until tender.
3. Divide the sweet potato, arugula, quinoa, black beans, tomatoes, carrots, avocado, and hemp seeds evenly between 2 bowls and/or storage containers. When you're ready to serve, squeeze a fresh lemon half over each bowl, and enjoy.
4. Store leftovers in the refrigerator for up to 3 days.

Kitchen Tip: If you are making this for meal prep, be sure to let all of the ingredients cool completely before you assemble the bowls, so you don't wilt the greens and raw veggies.

Shortcut: It's easy to make a bowl like this at the salad bar! Start with a generous portion of greens, then add lots of your favorite raw veggies; a protein such as a hard-boiled egg, ½ cup of baked tofu, or 3 ounces of grilled chicken (stick to that palm-size portion); a small serving of avocado or nuts; and a healthy carb like fruit or quinoa. Top with 1 tablespoon of dressing and smile at the knowledge that you're sticking to your plan!

Prep time: 15 minutes
Cook time: 15 minutes
Makes: 2 bowls
Serving size: 1 bowl

Greek Power Bowl with Shrimp

Recharge your day with this power bowl! The Mediterranean diet is so good for your heart and overall health, and this recipe checks all of the boxes with savory shrimp, lots of fresh veggies, briny olives, and creamy feta cheese.

2 teaspoons olive oil, divided
3 ounces medium shrimp, peeled and deveined, thawed if frozen
½ teaspoon dried oregano
1 cup arugula
½ cup canned chickpeas, rinsed and drained
¼ cup halved grape tomatoes
¼ of a cucumber, chopped
2 tablespoons finely chopped red onion
2 tablespoons crumbled feta cheese
5 pitted kalamata olives, halved
Fresh dill, for garnish (optional)
1 tablespoon lemon juice
Salt and freshly ground pepper

1. Heat 1 teaspoon of the olive oil in a medium sauté pan over medium-high heat. Add the shrimp and season with the oregano and salt and pepper. Cook until the shrimp are pink and opaque, stirring occasionally, about 4 minutes. Set aside.
2. Add the arugula to a large bowl and top with the chickpeas, tomatoes, cucumber, red onion, feta, olives, and dill (if using).
3. Top with the shrimp, drizzle with the lemon juice and the remaining teaspoon of olive oil, and serve.

Prep time: 10 minutes
Cook time: 5 minutes
Makes: 1 bowl | Serving size: 1 bowl

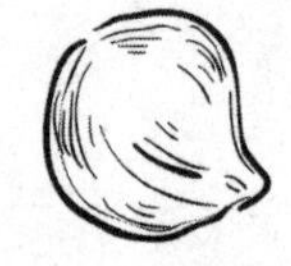
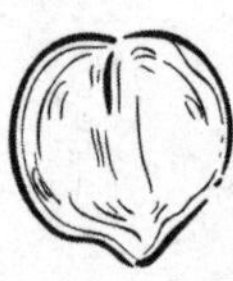

Feta and Spinach Salmon Salad

This hearty salad is super filling and meal-prep friendly! You'll be feeling strong and healthy after a large bowl of spinach topped with heart-healthy salmon. Make a double batch if you want to enjoy it twice.

For the salad:

1 teaspoon extra-virgin olive oil
1 (3-ounce) salmon fillet, skin on
¼ cup chopped red onion
2 cups baby spinach
¼ cup diced yellow bell pepper
2 tablespoons crumbled feta cheese
Salt and freshly ground pepper

For the dressing:

½ teaspoon lemon zest
1 tablespoon fresh lemon juice
1 tablespoon balsamic vinegar
1 clove garlic, minced
1 teaspoon Dijon mustard
1 teaspoon olive oil

1. Heat a medium nonstick pan over medium-high heat with 1 teaspoon of olive oil. Season the salmon with a pinch of salt and pepper and cook, skin side down, for 3 to 4 minutes. Add the onion to the pan, reduce the heat to medium, cover, and continue to cook until the onion is wilted and the salmon is cooked to your liking, about 1 to 2 minutes more.
2. Combine the spinach, bell pepper, and feta in a bowl.
3. In a small bowl, whisk together the lemon zest, lemon juice, vinegar, garlic, mustard, and olive oil.
4. Drizzle dressing over salad and top with the salmon and onion. Cheers!

Prep time: 10 minutes | Cook time: 10 minutes
Makes: 1 salad | Serving size: 1 salad

Dinner Recipes

Blueberry Balsamic Turkey Meatballs

Serve this meal at a party and impress all of your friends! This dish has so many unique ingredients that come together to form one wonderful recipe. Who knew blueberries and balsamic vinegar would be such a great combo?

For the sauce:

2 cups fresh or frozen blueberries
¼ cup balsamic vinegar
2 tablespoons all-fruit grape jelly
1½ tablespoons honey
½ teaspoon garlic powder
½ teaspoon salt

For the meatballs:

12 ounces 99% lean ground turkey
¼ cup finely chopped cilantro
¼ cup finely chopped onion
1 egg, lightly beaten
2 cloves garlic, minced
1 teaspoon chili powder
Salt and freshly ground pepper

For serving:

1 cup cooked brown rice

1. In a blender or food processor, process the blueberries, balsamic vinegar, grape jelly, honey, garlic powder, and salt until smooth.
2. Transfer the blueberry mixture to a small saucepan. Bring to a boil, then reduce heat and simmer for 10 minutes. Set aside.
3. To prepare the meatballs, use your hands to combine the ground turkey, cilantro, onion, egg, garlic, chili powder, and a pinch of salt and pepper.
4. Use your hands to shape the meatballs into 12 equal-size balls.

5. Heat a large nonstick skillet over medium heat. Lightly coat the skillet with cooking spray, then add the meatballs and cook, turning twice to ensure all sides are browned, around 7 minutes.
6. Pour the blueberry mixture over the meatballs, cover, and simmer for 10 minutes.
7. Divide the brown rice between four serving bowls and/or storage containers, top each serving with three meatballs, and drizzle excess sauce over each bowl.
8. Store leftovers in the refrigerator for up to 3 days or freeze individual portions for up to 3 months. To reheat, defrost in refrigerator overnight (if frozen) and microwave on high for 4 minutes, or until heated through.

Prep time: 10 minutes | Cook time: 20 minutes
Makes: 12 meatballs | Serving size: 3 meatballs plus ¼ of sauce

Greek Turkey Burgers

Ground turkey is so much leaner than beef, so this blended burger gives you all of the burger satisfaction with less fat. Creamy yogurt-feta sauce tops a pita packed with all of the crunchy veggies for a quick and delicious dinner that can also be made in advance. Try this one at your next barbecue!

For the burger:

½ cup canned chickpeas, drained and rinsed
4 ounces 99% lean ground turkey
¼ cup finely chopped yellow onion
1 clove garlic, minced
½ teaspoon dried oregano
1 teaspoon lemon zest
1 teaspoon olive oil
Salt and freshly ground pepper

For the yogurt-feta sauce:

¼ cup unsweetened nonfat Greek yogurt
2 tablespoons crumbled feta
1 tablespoon lemon juice
1 tablespoon fresh mint, finely chopped
1 tablespoon fresh dill, finely chopped (or 1 teaspoon dried)
5 pitted kalamata olives, finely chopped
1 clove garlic, minced

To serve:

1 whole wheat pita, halved
1 cup quartered grape tomatoes
1 cup diced cucumber
½ cup thinly sliced red bell pepper

1. In a large bowl, crush the chickpeas with a potato masher or the bottom of a drinking glass. Add the ground turkey, onion, garlic, oregano, lemon zest, olive oil, and a pinch of salt and pepper. Use your hands to shape the mixture into 2 (4-inch) patties.
2. Heat a grill or grill pan over medium-high heat. Place patties over the grill and cook 5 minutes on each side.

3. While the burgers are cooking, stir the yogurt, feta, lemon juice, mint, dill, olives, and garlic together in a small bowl. Set aside.
4. To serve, fill one pita half with a burger, half of the tomatoes, cucumber, and peppers, and half of the sauce. Serve immediately.

Kitchen Tip: This recipe makes 2 burgers, so plan to have the other burger for lunch during the week. Store the burger, sauce, and chopped veggies separately in airtight containers for up to 5 days (divided containers work great here). Heat burger on a microwave-safe plate for 2 minutes, or until heated through, then pile burger, toppings, and sauce into the pita and enjoy.

Prep time: 10 minutesCook time: 10 minutes
Makes: 2 burgers
Serving size: 1 burger

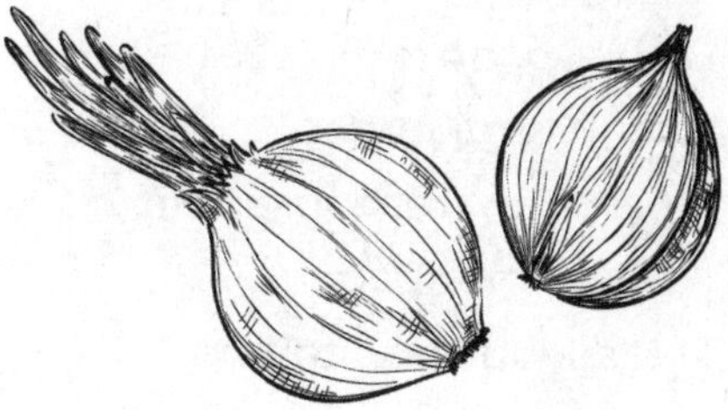

Lemon-Herb Chicken Pasta

How about a big plate of pasta in a light sauce with lemony chicken and lots of green vegetables? The trick here is to reserve some of the pasta cooking water—it will blend with the lemon marinade and Parmesan, allowing the flavors of the pasta and veggies to shine through.

4 ounces whole wheat penne
1 boneless, skinless chicken breast (about ½ pound)
2 tablespoons extra-virgin olive oil, divided
1 tablespoon lemon zest
Juice from 1 lemon
1 teaspoon fresh rosemary, finely chopped
1 teaspoon fresh thyme, minced
3 cloves garlic, minced, divided
1 medium red onion, halved and thinly sliced
1 cup sliced button mushrooms
1 medium zucchini, diced
½ cup fresh or frozen peas
2 cups baby spinach
¼ cup grated Parmesan cheese
Salt and freshly ground pepper

1. Bring a 3-quart saucepan of water to a boil. Add a large pinch of salt, then cook the pasta until al dente, about 12 minutes. Reserve ½ cup of cooking water; then drain the pasta and set aside.
2. While the pasta is cooking, cut the chicken into bite-size chunks. Whisk 1 tablespoon of the olive oil with the lemon zest and juice, rosemary, thyme, and 1 clove minced garlic. Stir in the chicken and season with salt and pepper. Cover and refrigerate until needed.
3. Heat the remaining tablespoon of olive oil in a large sauté pan over medium-high heat. Add the remaining 2 cloves of garlic, onion, and mushrooms, and sauté until the mushrooms begin to brown, about 5 minutes. Season with salt and pepper.

4. Add the chicken and marinade, then stir to scrape up any browned bits stuck to the bottom of the pan. Add reserved pasta cooking water, cover, and cook for 5 minutes.
5. Stir in the zucchini, peas, and pasta, and cook for 2 minutes more. Add the spinach and continue to stir until the spinach is just wilted, about 1 minute. Add the Parmesan, stir to combine, and serve immediately.
6. Leftovers can be stored for up to 3 days in the fridge. To reheat, place pasta in a microwave-safe dish, drizzle with 1 tablespoon of water, and cover with a damp paper towel. Heat for 2 minutes, stir, then heat for 1 minute more, or until hot.

Kitchen Tip: If you can't imagine pasta without tomato sauce, go ahead and stir in ½ cup of your favorite jarred marinara when you add the zucchini, pasta, and peas.

Prep time: 10 minutes
Cook time: 30 minutes
Makes 2 servings
Serving size: ½ of pasta

Sheet Pan Shrimp and Broccoli

Throw this easy sheet pan meal together on a busy evening. Lemony garlic shrimp cooks up on the same pan as broccoli and fingerling potatoes—this super-simple dinner is high on flavor and low on dishes! Save the second serving for another meal or share it with someone special.

4 cups fresh broccoli florets
6 ounces small fingerling potatoes, quartered (about 6 potatoes)
2 tablespoons olive oil, divided
1 teaspoon lemon zest
1 tablespoon fresh lemon juice
2 cloves garlic, minced
10 ounces medium shrimp, peeled and deveined
Pinch crushed red pepper flakes
Salt and freshly ground pepper

1. Heat oven to 400°F. Line a large, rimmed baking sheet with parchment paper.
2. Toss the broccoli and fingerling potatoes on the baking sheet with 1 tablespoon of the olive oil. Spread the vegetables in an even layer and season lightly with salt and pepper. Roast for 15 minutes.
3. Meanwhile, whisk the remaining tablespoon of olive oil, lemon zest, lemon juice, and garlic in a medium bowl. Stir in the shrimp; season with crushed red pepper flakes, salt, and pepper; and set aside.
4. Remove the broccoli and potatoes from the oven, stir, and add the shrimp and marinade. Spread everything out into an even layer, then return to the oven for 10 minutes. Serve immediately. Leftovers can be stored in an airtight container in the fridge for up to 3 days. To reheat, place on a microwave-safe dish and microwave for 2 minutes or until heated through.

Prep time: 10 minutes | Cook time: 25 minutes
Makes: 2 servings | Serving size: ½ of recipe

Teriyaki Tuna with Roasted Green Beans and Soba

Soba are delicious Japanese buckwheat noodles that are great served hot or cold—here, they're served in a chilled salad with roasted green beans and a flavorful teriyaki tuna.

For tuna and green beans:

2 tablespoons low-sodium soy sauce
2 tablespoons rice vinegar
2 tablespoons honey
1 teaspoon lemon juice
2 teaspoons sesame seeds
2 (4-ounce) tuna steaks
6 ounces green beans, trimmed
1 tablespoon olive oil
Salt and freshly ground pepper

For soba salad:

1 bundle soba noodles
1 medium carrot, shredded or spiralized
1 medium zucchini, shredded or spiralized
1 teaspoon toasted sesame oil
1 teaspoon rice vinegar
1 tablespoon nori furikake (see Kitchen Tip below)

1. Preheat oven to 450°F. Bring a medium saucepan of water to a boil.
2. In a large bowl, mix the soy sauce, rice vinegar, honey, lemon juice, and sesame seeds and whisk until well combined.
3. Add the tuna to the marinade, cover, and marinate in the refrigerator for at least 15 minutes (or up to 8 hours).
4. Add 1 bundle of soba noodles to the boiling water and cook according to package directions. Drain, rinse well with cold water, and set aside.
5. On a large, rimmed baking sheet, toss the green beans with the olive oil. Season with salt and pepper and roast for 10 minutes, stirring once.
6. Add the tuna to the sheet pan (discarding the marinade) and return to the oven for 2 minutes. Flip the tuna and cook for 1

minute more for medium-rare, or 2 minutes (or longer) if you prefer it fully cooked.

7. Toss the soba noodles with the carrot, zucchini, sesame oil, rice vinegar, and nori furikake. Serve half of the noodle salad and green beans with 1 tuna steak. Leftovers will keep in the fridge for up to 3 days. Serve leftovers cold—tuna becomes "fishy" when overcooked or reheated!

Kitchen Tip: Nori furikake is a savory seasoning mix made of seaweed (nori), sesame seeds, and spices. It's easy to find at any Asian market. If you're in a pinch, slice roasted nori strips from the snack department of your supermarket into thin strips and mix into the salad with a teaspoon of sesame seeds.

Prep time: 10 minutes | Cook time: 20 minutes
Makes: 2 servings | Serving size: 1 tuna steak plus ½ of salad

Veggie Pizza with Cauliflower Crust

Sometimes you just need a pizza, and nothing else will do! Here's one you can indulge in without any guilt! Once you've got the hang of it, mix things up with your favorite veggie toppings.

- 1 cauliflower head, stemmed and cut into small florets
- 1 tablespoon olive oil, divided
- 2 large eggs
- 2 tablespoons grated Parmesan cheese
- 2 cloves garlic, minced
- ½ cup white button mushrooms, sliced
- ½ yellow onion, thinly sliced
- ½ cup zucchini, thinly sliced
- ½ cup yellow bell pepper, thinly sliced
- 1 (14.5-ounce) can plum tomatoes, drained and roughly chopped
- ½ teaspoon dried oregano
- 2 tablespoons chopped kalamata olives
- 1 cup baby spinach
- ½ cup shredded mozzarella cheese
- Salt and freshly ground pepper

For serving:

Handful of fresh basil leaves

1. Preheat oven to 400°F. Spray a large, rimmed baking sheet with cooking spray.
2. To make the crust, steam the cauliflower florets until tender (or microwave for 4–5 minutes with a few tablespoons of water). Drain, then pulse in a blender or food processor until it reaches a smooth consistency—it should look like fluffy rice. Cool slightly, then use a clean kitchen towel to squeeze all the excess liquid from the cauliflower. (This step is essential to the success of your cauliflower crust—don't skip it!)

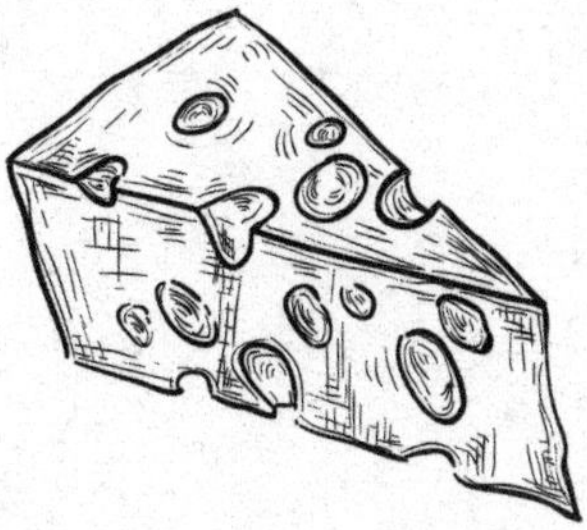

3. Combine the cauliflower, 1 teaspoon of the olive oil, eggs, Parmesan, garlic, and a generous pinch of salt and pepper in a large bowl. Mix well to combine.
4. Using your hands, press the cauliflower mixture into 2 (8-inch diameter) circles on the prepared baking sheet.
5. Coat the crusts with 1 teaspoon of the olive oil and bake for about 25 minutes.
6. Heat a medium saucepan over medium-high heat. Add the remaining teaspoon of olive oil to the pan and swirl to coat. Add the mushrooms, onion, zucchini, and bell pepper, and sauté until tender. Add the tomatoes, oregano, and olives and stir for 5 minutes.
7. Top each baked crust with half of the veggie/tomato mixture, half of the baby spinach, and half of the mozzarella. Return to the oven and bake for 10 minutes more, or until the cheese is melted and beginning to brown. Top with the basil leaves and serve immediately.

Note: Once you've baked the cauliflower crust, you can cool it completely, wrap it tightly in plastic wrap, and store it in the freezer for 2 months. Defrost for about 20 minutes before topping, then bake for about 15 minutes, or until the cheese is melted and everything is bubbling hot. Store the second portion of sauce in an airtight container in the freezer; defrost in refrigerator before using.

Shortcut: Whole wheat pitas make a great single-serving pizza. Simply drizzle with a little olive oil, top with the veggie sauce and cheese, and bake for 10 minutes.

Prep time: 20 minutes | Cook time: 45 minutes
Makes: 2 pizzas | Serving size: 1 pizza

Spaghetti Squash with Tomato Sauce and Cod

Who doesn't love spaghetti? Spaghetti squash is a healthy, lower-carb alternative that's full of fiber and nutrients. Topped with flaky cod in in a flavorful tomato sauce, this meal is affordable, nutritious, and delicious!

1 small spaghetti squash
1 tablespoon olive oil, divided
3 cloves garlic, minced
1 small yellow onion, finely chopped
1 cup sliced white button mushrooms
½ cup finely chopped celery
1 (14.5-ounce) can plum tomatoes, with liquid, lightly crushed by hand
1 teaspoon Italian seasoning blend (or a mix of oregano and thyme)
2 (4-ounce) cod fillets (pin bones removed, if necessary)
¾ cup thinly sliced fresh basil
Salt and freshly ground pepper

1. Preheat oven to 400°F.
2. With a sharp knife, cut the top and bottom edges off the squash, then carefully cut it in half lengthwise. Use a spoon to scoop out the seeds, then coat the inside of the squash with 1 teaspoon of the olive oil. On a large, rimmed baking sheet lined with parchment paper, bake the squash cut-side down for 45 to 50 minutes, or until the squash is tender and cut sides are turning golden brown. Set aside to cool.
3. Once squash is cool enough to handle, use a fork to scrape the inside, creating spaghetti-like strands. Set aside.
4. While the squash is cooling, heat the remaining 2 teaspoons of olive oil in a large sauté pan over medium heat. Add the garlic, onion, mushrooms, and celery, and sauté until the onion is softened and the mushrooms are beginning to brown, about 5

minutes. Add the tomatoes and Italian seasoning blend, season with salt and pepper to taste, and bring to a simmer. Carefully add the cod fillets. Reduce the heat to medium-low, cover, and cook, stirring once or twice, for 10 minutes, or until the cod is opaque and flakes easily with a fork.

5. To serve, divide the spaghetti squash between two in bowls and/or storage containers. Top each with 1 cod fillet and half of the sauce. Garnish each serving with a large handful of basil and a little freshly ground pepper. Store leftovers in an airtight container in the fridge for up to 3 days or in the freezer for up to 3 months. Reheat in the microwave, 1 minute at a time, stirring frequently until heated through.

Kitchen Tip: If you like it spicy, stir in some crushed red pepper flakes when you add the tomatoes. You can make this dish with shrimp, too—they'll only need 5 minutes of cooking time once you've added them to the tomato sauce.

Prep time: 15 minutes | Cook time: 65 minutes
Makes: 2 servings | Serving size: 1 cod fillet plus ½ of squash and sauce

Light Tofu Thai Curry

Curry is a unique spice mixture that transforms a recipe. There are three traditional Thai curry styles—green, red, and yellow. This recipe calls for green curry, which is the sweetest of the three. Look for small jars in the Asian aisle at your supermarket—you don't want to skip this ingredient.

1 (16-ounce) package extra-firm tofu
2 tablespoons coconut oil, divided
1 bunch asparagus, trimmed and cut into 2-inch pieces
2 cups green beans, trimmed and cut into 2-inch pieces
1 yellow onion, halved and thinly sliced
1 yellow bell pepper, seeded and thinly sliced
2 tablespoons Thai green curry paste
1 (14.5-ounce) can light coconut milk
1 tablespoon soy sauce
2 teaspoons honey
1 tablespoon fresh lime juice
2 teaspoons lime zest

For serving:
1 cup cooked brown rice
½ cup cilantro
Handful fresh basil leaves

1. Drain the liquid from the tofu, then wrap it in a clean kitchen towel and place it on a cutting board with a heavy object (like a thick cookbook) on top to press out the extra moisture. Allow it to sit for 15 to 20 minutes. Cut tofu into 1-inch cubes.
2. Heat 1 tablespoon of the coconut oil in a large nonstick skillet over medium-high heat. Add the tofu and sauté for 5 minutes, or until lightly browned, stirring occasionally. Drain the tofu and set it aside.
3. Heat the remaining tablespoon of coconut oil over medium-high heat in the same pan. Add the asparagus, green beans, onion, and bell pepper; sauté for 4 minutes. Stir in the curry paste. Add the

coconut milk, soy sauce, honey, lime juice, and lime zest, and stir to combine.

4. Return the tofu to the pan, bring to a simmer, and cook until the vegetables are tender and the sauce has thickened slightly, about 3 minutes more.
5. Divide the cooked rice evenly between three bowls and/or storage containers; then top each with the tofu and vegetable mixture. Garnish with cilantro and basil. Store leftovers in an airtight container in the refrigerator for up to 5 days or freeze for up to 2 months. To reheat from frozen, defrost overnight in the refrigerator, then microwave for about 5 minutes or until heated through.

Kitchen Tip: When you're meal prepping, get your tofu pressed and proteins marinating, then do other prep work in the meantime. The more you prep, the more you'll find that it's easy to save time by prepping more than one recipe/food at a time.

Prep time: 25 minutes
Cook time: 15 minutes
Makes: 3 servings
Serving size: ⅓ of curry and rice

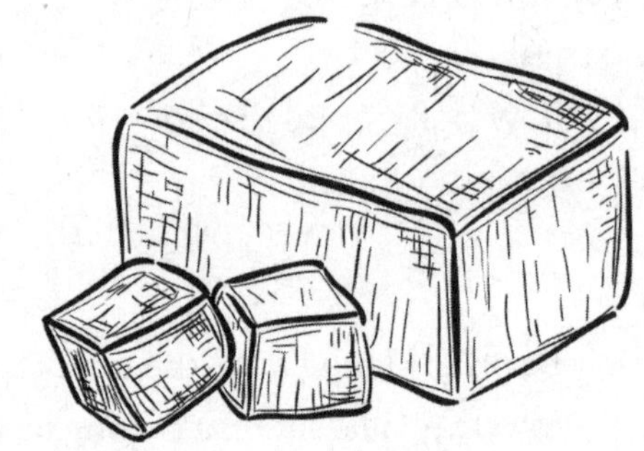

Halibut and Veggie Skewers

It's hard to beat a grilled, well-balanced skewer! This recipe is packed with omega 3, healthy fats, veggies, complex carbs, and protein—making it an all-around balanced meal.

For the marinade:
½ cup chopped basil
1 small shallot, finely chopped
2 tablespoons extra-virgin olive oil
2 tablespoons lemon juice
1 clove garlic, minced
Pinch crushed red pepper flakes
Salt and freshly ground pepper

For the skewers:
10 ounces halibut, cut into cubes
1 zucchini, halved lengthwise and cut into 1½-inch-thick slices
1 yellow onion, cut into wedges
1 (14-ounce) can water-packed artichoke hearts, drained
1 lemon, thinly sliced

To serve:
2 cups arugula
½ cup halved grape tomatoes

1. To prepare the marinade, combine the basil, shallot, olive oil, lemon juice, garlic, and red pepper flakes in a blender or food processor and process until well combined. Season with salt and pepper, pulse once more, and divide into two bowls, one for brushing the fish and one for serving. Set aside.
2. Carefully thread the halibut, zucchini, onions, artichokes, and lemon slices alternately onto 4 skewers. (I like to use metal skewers—if you're using wooden skewers, be sure to soak them in water first.) Brush on most of one bowl of the marinade to coat the skewers.
3. Heat a grill or grill pan to medium-high heat, spray generously with cooking spray, and cook the skewers for 6 minutes, turning

once, or until the halibut is opaque and firm to the touch. Brush with a little more marinade after turning. (Alternately, broil in the oven at the highest setting and rack position for about 3 minutes per side.)

4. Drizzle the arugula and tomatoes with the reserved marinade. Divide between 2 plates and/or storage containers, with half of the arugula salad and 2 skewers per serving. Store arugula and tomatoes in a separate container. Enjoy the second portion of halibut skewers cold, or reheat in microwave for about 2 minutes, or just until heated through.

Prep time: 10 minutes | Cook time: 10 minutes
Makes: 2 servings | Serving size: ½ of arugula salad and 2 skewers

Lemon Parmesan Salmon Zoodles

This balanced meal is perfectly proportioned, with a large portion of veggies, a palm-size serving of protein, and a zesty lemon flavor that will wake up your taste buds! This meal is one of my favorites to cook at summer gatherings; I'm sure your guests will love it, too.

2 teaspoons olive oil, divided
2 (4-ounce) salmon fillets
2 large zucchini, spiralized
1 tablespoon butter or ghee
3 cloves garlic, minced
2 teaspoons chopped fresh thyme
1 teaspoon chopped fresh rosemary
2 teaspoons lemon zest
⅔ cup vegetable broth
¼ cup grated Parmesan cheese
Salt and freshly ground pepper

To serve:
Lemon slices

1. Heat 1 teaspoon of the olive oil in a 12-inch sauté pan over medium heat. Season the salmon with salt and pepper and cook skin-side down for about 4 minutes, then flip and cook for 1 minute more. Remove the salmon from the pan and set aside. Carefully wipe the pan clean.
2. Heat the remaining teaspoon of olive oil over medium heat in the same skillet. Once the oil is hot, add the zucchini and sauté for 3 minutes, or until just tender. Remove the zucchini from the pan and set aside.
3. Add the butter, garlic, thyme, rosemary, and lemon zest to the pan. Stir for 1 minute, then add the vegetable broth and increase the heat to medium-high to bring the sauce to a boil.
4. Stir in the Parmesan, reduce heat to low, and simmer for 3 minutes, or until the sauce starts to thicken up.
5. Layer the salmon on top of the zucchini noodles, pour the sauce over everything, garnish with lemon slices, and serve

immediately. Store leftovers in an airtight container in the fridge for up to 3 days. Be gentle when reheating salmon—it will become "fishy" if overcooked. Start with 2 minutes and stir gently. Microwave until just heated through, or simmer in a covered saucepan over low heat if you prefer.

Shortcut: If you don't have a spiralizer or you're short on time, look for premade "zoodles" in your supermarket's produce department.

Prep time: 10 minutes | Cook time: 20 minutes
Makes: 2 servings | Serving size: ½ of zoodles plus 1 salmon fillet

APPENDIX A

Meal Prep Recipes and Tips

Meal prep doesn't have to be a chore—approach it with an organized mindset and the realization that you are taking great care of your health, and you will soon begin to look forward to your meal-prep sessions. Plan your menu (or use the menu plan in this book), shop for your groceries, put on your favorite music, and get cooking!

Meal-Prep Tricks and Tips

First things first. Identify the items you'll need in several recipes and make those first. It's easy to make one batch of brown rice, quinoa, or hard-boiled eggs, and then just grab them as you need them.

Hard-boiled eggs: Place your eggs in a saucepan, add water to cover by 2 inches, and bring to a boil. Cover the pan, turn off the heat, and set a timer for exactly 10 minutes. Remove the eggs with a slotted spoon to a bowl filled with ice water, then drain and refrigerate. Store in the fridge for up to 1 week.

Brown rice: Rinse 1 cup of brown rice in a strainer until the water runs clear. Place it in a small saucepan with 1¾ cups water and a pinch of salt. Bring to a boil, stir once (and once only), then cover, reduce heat to the lowest setting, and set a timer for 45 minutes (or set timer according to package directions—some varieties take more or less time). At the end of the cooking time, turn off the heat and let stand, covered, for 5 minutes. Cool completely and store in the fridge for up to 4 days, or in the freezer in individual ½ cup portions for up to 3 months. To reheat rice, place in a microwave-safe bowl and cover with a damp paper towel. Microwave until hot, about 90 seconds for refrigerated rice or 2 minutes for frozen.

Quinoa: Quinoa contains a mild toxin called *saponin* that helps the plant defend itself from predators. It can be bitter and soapy tasting, and may even give you a tummy ache, so it's essential to rinse quinoa well, even if the package says "pre-rinsed." Rinse 1 cup of quinoa under plenty of running water until it's no longer foamy. Place it in a small saucepan with 1¾ cups water and a pinch of salt. Bring to a boil, stir once, then cover and reduce heat to low. Cook for 15 minutes, then turn off the heat and let it stand, covered, for 5 minutes more. Follow storage and reheating instructions for brown rice above.

Invite a friend. Meal prep can be daunting when you're first starting out, so why not get a friend to do it with you? Prepping doesn't have to be a chore. You can make it a meal-prep party! Double the recipes, and take turns cooking and washing dishes. At the end of the day, you'll have healthy meals ready to go and you had a great time doing it. If your kitchen is too tiny for two, split up the work, then get together for a cup of tea and a meal-prep exchange.

Find your routine. The meal prep in this book has been organized to do two prep sessions per week, with a few meals cooked fresh (some, like smoothies, have to be made on the spot). You'll quickly find what works for you. Maybe you want to spend a few hours on a Sunday cooking up all of your meals and loading up the freezer, or maybe you like to come home from work each evening and enjoy the ritual of cooking dinner. And if you want to drink the same smoothie for breakfast every day, that's your choice; however, I encourage you to take this month to try some new things—you may find a new favorite or two!

Be prepared. Shopping and prepping on the same day can be tiring, so you might want to shop the day before you prep your meals. Before you begin, read through the recipes so you know what to expect. Get out your equipment, fill up your water bottle, put on some music, and get ready to cook!

Keep it fresh. The recipes in this book have storage suggestions for refrigerating and, when appropriate, freezing your meals. Some foods are great when made in advance, and some are better cooked fresh. Consider, for instance, buying and preparing perishables, such as fish, the day you're planning to cook them for maximum flavor and quality.

Clean as you go. Trust me—you don't want to wait until the end of your prep day to start doing the dishes. Clean up as you go, and you'll be organized and focused. Let it all pile up, and you'll quickly find yourself overwhelmed and vowing to eat takeout for the rest of your life.

Be okay with mistakes. In most cases, even if you've messed up, it's still going to be edible. Cooking nutritious food for yourself is one of the best forms of self-care you can practice, and learning to do it is a process! Relax and embrace (and eat) your mistakes, and you'll learn how to make it better next time.

Safety first. Use a sharp knife and a clean cutting board—you're much more likely to cut yourself with a dull knife than a sharp one. If you don't have good knife skills, watch a YouTube video to learn how to properly slice and dice. And if the only knife in your kitchen is a rusty old steak knife, do yourself a favor and buy a proper chef's knife and paring knife. You can't do the job if you don't have the proper tools, and you don't have to spend big bucks to buy a quality knife.

Have fun! You deserve to feed your body wholesome, nutritious food. If you don't do this for yourself, no one is going to do it for you. Like any skill, meal prep gets easier with time, so learn as you go, and soon you'll be loving every minute of it.

APPENDIX B

Tips for Freezing Foods

The freezer is your best friend when you're eating home-cooked meals every day. Use these tips to keep your food at its best quality when you're storing it in the freezer.

- Use only freezer-safe, BPA-free plastic or glass.
- Cool foods completely before storing—never put hot foods directly into the freezer.
- Leave 1 inch of "headspace" at the top of each container. Food expands when you freeze it, so if you fill the container all the way to the top, the lid will pop off and your food will get freezer burn.
- When storing small items like No-Bake Lime Coconut Protein Bites (page 249) or Blueberry Greek Yogurt Pancakes (page 237), freeze them individually on a sheet pan or plate first, then transfer to a freezer-safe storage bag once they're completely frozen.

- To store egg dishes like breakfast bakes and frittatas, cool completely, then wrap each individual portion in plastic wrap, and place multiple servings in a freezer-safe plastic bag to grab as you need them.
- Avoid freezing potatoes, dairy products, and watery vegetables like lettuce.
- Defrost meals and casseroles in the fridge overnight for best results. If you forget, you can use the "defrost" setting on your microwave. Egg dishes, pancakes, and rice/quinoa can be reheated directly from the freezer.
- Wrap items securely and label them with the date you put them in the freezer.
- Before you eat something from the freezer, check it for quality. Look for freezer burn or ice crystals. If it's been in there too long, or you've had a power outage that lasted more than twenty-four hours, you know what to do. When in doubt, throw it out!

Index

Recipe Index

Z

About the Author

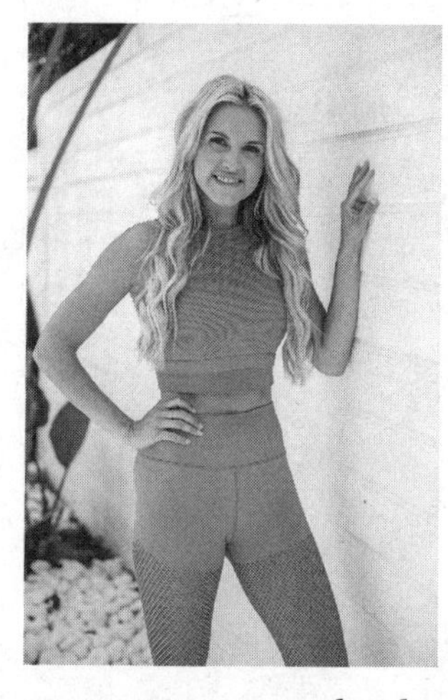

Originally from the United Kingdom, **REBECCA LOUISE** came to the United States at age twenty-three on a whim to get her commercial pilot's license, which she completed out of the Long Beach, California, airport. The small-town girl from Eastbourne, England, had grown up watching MTV's *The Hills*, and after landing at LAX, she knew that this is where she was meant to be. Rebecca played field hockey for the South of England and participated in many sports teams at school; she is also a trained dancer. After struggling with anorexia at age seventeen and being bullied throughout school, she never let anything stop her from following her dreams. Although Rebecca loved flying, it was not her ultimate passion. After obtaining her work visa to come to the States, she was cast on a fitness YouTube channel, where Rebecca's love for fitness, helping people, and hosting came alive. Since then, her YouTube views have surpassed more than 450 million, and Rebecca went on to create her fitness and nutrition app, BURN. Rebecca lives in Huntington Beach with her two dogs,

Alphie and Pennie. She has traveled to more than twenty countries to host fit camps to meet her fans and help them feel the BURN! Her podcast, *It Takes Grit*, launched in January 2019 and is already in the top charts in some countries. The purpose of the podcast is to inspire and give others the plan to take action. Rebecca's programs have been featured in *Entrepreneur*, *Vogue*, *Allure*, *Cosmopolitan*, and *Shape*, and on KTLA, Fox, Oxygen, Closer Weekly, Well+Good, and Goop.com.